Yoga

Learn Yoga Poses to Calm the Mind, Relieve Stress, Strengthen the Body, and Increase Flexibility

(Essential Essentials Yoga Workout Book to Recover From Arthritis, and Achieve Weight Loss)

Dianne Baptiste

Published by Rob Miles

Dianne Baptiste

Yoga: Learn Yoga Poses to Calm the Mind, Relieve Stress, Strengthen the Body, and Increase Flexibility (Essential Essentials Yoga Workout Book to Recover From Arthritis, and Achieve Weight Loss)

ISBN 978-1-989990-58-2

Legal & Disclaimer

The information contained in this book is not designed to replace or take the place of any form of medicine or professional medical advice. The information in this book has been provided for educational and entertainment purposes only.

The information contained in this book has been compiled from sources deemed reliable, and it is accurate to the best of the Author's knowledge; however, the Author cannot guarantee its accuracy and validity and cannot be held liable for any errors or omissions. Changes are periodically made to this book. You must consult your doctor or get professional medical advice before using any of the suggested remedies, techniques, or information in this book.

Table of Contents

Yoga brings you back home, to your True Self, where everything is good. With many schools and principles in practice now, Yoga has emerged from being a beautiful poetic composition that blends physical, mental, and spiritual aspects into yet another form of exercise. If you take a close look at the actual practice of Yoga, you will realize that its physical part is only meant to help you take a deeper plunge into your spiritual life.

Yin Yoga is a softer side of Yoga. It doesn't contain strenuous Vinyasa flows like your Ashtanga or Power Yoga classes. Yet, it gifts you a mesmerizing dose of flexibility and strength.

At the end of a session your mat will be clean, free from the stink of your sweat. You will not find yourself in difficult arm balances and inversions. You will find yourself practicing seated Asanas, or the poses. Very rarely, you will do a Dangling Doll or a Downward Facing Dog.

Yet it is a beautiful yoga style that is well-known for its restorative benefits – physically, mentally, and spiritually. Ideally, this style would lead you towards greater physical, mental, and spiritual health. It restores the natural functioning of the body while rendering mental steadiness. Further, these Asanas help heal our physical, mental, and spiritual imbalances.

The focus is more on breath, and the intention is to let go. As you move from one asana to the next, there are no jerks or jumps. The movements are fluid and soft. You do not force yourself or hyper-extend your body. You just allow it to be in its natural state, allowing your breath to do rest of the work.

The modern day Yoga sessions have been built upon classical Hatha. But in this transformation, Yoga lost some of its valuable elements. The focus is more on a muscular level while you often tend to overlook the underlying soft tissues, including cartilages, joints, and ligaments.

Yin Yoga will bring your focus to these forgotten body parts. It allows you to re-establish the lost connection among your body, mind, and soul.

It teaches you to breathe consciously. You are breathing, but most of the time involuntarily. Your breath doesn't reach your abdomen or chest. When you practice Yin Yoga, you will become more conscious of your breath.

The appropriate combination of breath and physical movements ease the conflicts experienced by your body and mind, enhancing your health.

Anyone can practice Yin Yoga. It doesn't matter if you practice an energetic style of yoga or any other workout. It doesn't matter if you are a beginner or novice. It doesn't matter if you are stiff or super flexible. Since the practice encourages the use of props like bolsters, straps, and blocks, you will be able to hold the postures for longer periods. And, slowly, you will find yourself enjoying benefits that you never experienced before.

And, that is what Yin Yoga teaches you! So, are you ready to rewrite your life a positive way? Are you ready for the change?

Let's get started! Best wishes!

Yoga is understood as being a process of marriage. This unification is multifaceted. In one single dimension, it is a marriage of the different systems which exist inside the human being such as religious, psychological, physical and intellectual. Altogether there are thought to be five distinct methods within human life. These are referred to as the koshas that are lively, the physical, psychological, delicate, and bliss sheaths. Within our current understanding of yoga, we're currently attempting to unify levels of the individual or these five figures. Another process of marriage occurs between the patient's consciousness and also the common consciousness.

This unification is often referred to as Samadhi and it is one of the primary transformations that arise inside the exercise of yoga. Observing this from the unique position, Samadhi can be a change of conception, which disillusionments concerning the world are reformed. Yoga can be stretched amongst different branches through which a person may pursue the progression and marriage of the elements inside their own bodies and minds. Each department retains a unique set of concepts and ideas which defines the final and process obtainment of complete unification.

There is no appropriate or inappropriate method of yoga because they each boast their distinctive traits that accommodate the needs of personalities and various qualities which exist among humans. Each technique is designed to provide another character type, and yoga is rolling out into a broad-reaching method that can be applied by almost anyone who's enthusiastic about living a religious life. Training like Jnana yoga is fantastic for a person who is philosophically minded while the exercise of bhakti yoga is not bad for a person who is emotionally intelligent and inclined towards a feeling of dedication.

Bhakti Yoga is the first process we shall examine. Bhakti yoga is just training when the psychic doctor focuses on having a state of loyalty within the center and the head. Together is expected to submit themselves through a method of self-surrendering to God, in bhakti yoga a powerful sense of belief is necessary.

Yoga's practice is usually based around one's Dharma or duties within the world. Dharma is determined by the patient in the past, including both pasts of the present lifestyle along with the pasts of previous lives. In a few values, Dharma will be the ultimate way for an individual since it is based on the practical sizes and potential of the person to utilize their time on earth for spiritual advance. One of the primary factors of Dharma is working on earth without the thought of the benefits or losses of the activities of one. The doctor lives and functions within the planet with no targets or enforced perceptions of how the future must distribute. The intellect employed by the advantage of the higher good in place of the separate desires of the average person and is concentrated on selfless service. In Karma yoga, the exercise is not steep since the individual slowly relinquishes the ties of juice and liberates the heart in the confines of egocentric thought processes.

The first mention of Juice yoga is at the Bhagavad-Gita in a talk between Krishna and Arjuna. Within this discussion, Krishna shows Arjuna that he could merge his mind with Krishna's when he surrenders his steps for the divine (which in cases like this is Krishna).

Kundalini Yoga Kundalini yoga is just a training of yoga which descends from the exercise of tantra yoga. One of the essential factors of tantra yoga is the increase of kundalini which will be considered to be the primordial pressure lifestyle within each human being. Control and the exercise of Kundalini yoga was formed to manage the potential of the kundalini power in the body. If not controlled while in the proper manner as the discharge of kundalini power can cause extreme physical and emotional disorders unlike other techniques of yoga, kundalini yoga could be a highly volatile practice of yoga.

Thus, the training of kundalini yoga is just a remarkably sophisticated process which is usually just practiced by those who find themselves properly advanced within the practices of spirituality. One of the primary conditions of kundalini yoga is a balanced body along with a powerful brain - without that, your launch of kundalini energy can be harmful if not deadly. A unique period in psychology known as kundalini syndrome continues to be developed for people who have gone into dementia because of kundalini energy's incorrect discharge. In yoga, the practices introduced are created to help wake the kundalini energy. Aside from its meaning while the primordial energy, Kundalini is also called the snake energy. At the platform of the backbone in the form of a spiraled coil similar to that of a serpent, the kundalini energy rests before its awareness. When produced, the kundalini energy shoots up through the backbone, producing its approach towards the crown of the pinnacle.

Hatha Yoga The word hatha has several definitions. Usually it is divided up into two specific terms, ha and tha. The meaning of these phrases can be viewed as the moon and the sunlight. It can also be said that these two phrases are sounds that are responsible for creating issue or Beeja Mantras. In the same time, ha represents the pranic body while tha is the fact of the mental body. Whichever model one decides to believe or follow, an important aspect of hatha yoga is a balancing of the polarities of power within the body (ida and pingala) along with a filter of your head and the body.

A lot of people, in a contemporary framework, consider hatha yoga to always be a training of the actual body. Although this is simply not improper, hatha yoga involves additional ideas and tactics that address more delicate features of the individual process. One of the primary factors of hatha yoga could be the aspect of purification. In hatha yoga filter occurs within the several factors of the person; a refinement is of the actual energetic, and emotional systems. It's assumed that once the bodies are all purified than religious development towards self-liberation may appear. Unlike Raja yoga, which we shall discuss later, hatha yoga does not summarize a prerequisite of moral values before doing yoga's methods. Instead, hatha yoga begins with the yoga postures or asanas and the lively refinement methods of pranayama.

Hatha yoga might be considered to be an initial exercise to more advanced systems of yoga, nonetheless it possesses within itself the capacity to guide towards spiritual freedom. A more moderate process of hatha yoga, of yoga can be applied to most of the people and doesn't require a well-established body-mind to start the training. Thus, it's a training employed by several who wish to use yoga an assistance towards spiritual independence.

Raja Yoga Raja Yoga is literally translated from Sanskrit as royal union and is the Noble course. Below, we are mainly worried about the standard method of Raja Yoga which has been applied considering the origins of the Sutras in India. Raja yoga is a route of psychic perception and also instinct. Thus those two features are expected to ensure that spiritual advancement to happen. Some spiritual masters like Swami Tureyananda genuinely believe that Raja yoga is used after considerable change has been received by one through initial methods of yoga.

Even a few other academics think that Raja yoga's practice is commenced after initial claims of Samadhi are not inexperienced. Consequently, Raja Yoga is not practice for the vast majority of people. In the yoga sutras, Patanjali carefully outlines the prerequisites for yoga's heightened techniques. The great majority of the yoga sutras are specialized in comprehension and managing the mind including its four pieces of Buddhi Chitta, Manas, and Ahamkara. Significant focus is directed at how the mind runs and works along with the various amounts and measurements that you can get to the brain. The rest of the writing discusses the stages through which one experience over the course towards self-realization, and awareness is directed at every one of the different traps that could happen along the way. Raja yoga's system is discussed and defined within the "8 limbed path."

CHAPTER 2: HOW DO YOU BEGIN?

While you can do yoga on your own, it is better that you find a trainer who will supervise and guide you. You will also gain more benefits from the practice if you will join classes, where you can hone camaraderie and friendship.

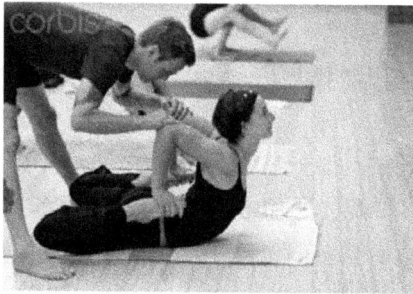

How do you find the right instructor and yoga class?

It is okay to ask a yoga instructor about his/her qualifications and experiences.

Let the instructor know why you are doing this.

Be open about your health condition. Talk to him/her about the body aches that you frequently suffer from. This way, he/she can design a yoga sequence that will not aggravate your condition.

Find a class that is suitable for beginners. Even when you think that you are strong enough to try the more difficult poses, it is better to begin with the simpler exercises that are easy to follow.

What are the styles of yoga that you can explore?

1. Ashtanga Yoga

This is athletic in nature. You will learn at your own pace and your teacher will help you in adjusting the movements depending on your strengths. The idea here is to observe and follow without rejecting anything. In life, this motivates you to keep on practicing because your mind is set that good things are coming.

2. Baptiste Power Vinyasa Yoga

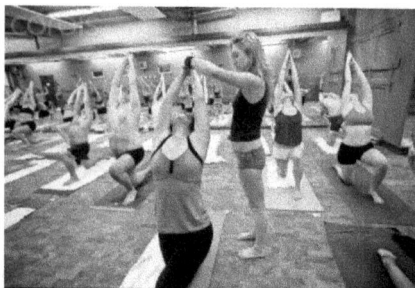

This is another physically demanding form of yoga. This is done in a heated room, where you will perform a vigorous sequence for 90 minutes. It helps you to cope with any challenges that may arise in the future. The goal of the exercises is to seek freedom and accept that you can become more powerful, live according to who you really are and have a peace of mind.

3. Bikram Yoga

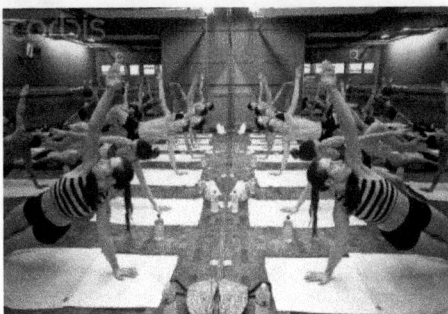

The classes are held in a heated room, where you will perform standing poses for 45 minutes and another 45 minutes doing floor postures. It aims to get your full mental concentration until you get to the point where your physical state is at one with your spiritual side. The movements will also make it easier for you to keep in shape and develop a great form.

4. Forrest Yoga

The practice requires strength. It actually helps you to celebrate your strength by releasing your emotional and physical tension. It helps you clean and clear your being from any baggage. This way, you are able to create enough room to welcome your spirit. This effectively combines tough physical activities with emotional exercises.

5. Integral Yoga

This involves gentle poses, meditation, chanting and breathing exercises. It pushes you to go back to your natural state, with a mind that is clear, a heart full of love and a life that is happy and contented.

6. Ishta Yoga

ISHTA means Integrated Science of Hatha, Tantra, and Ayurveda, a kind of yoga practice that balances the human organism in order to develop a stronger platform where you can easily attain spiritual growth. The movements that are involved in the practice are targeted to attain different kinds of energetic effects. It aligns your body, teaches you proper breathing techniques, hones your focus through meditation and cleanses your inner being.

7. Iyengar Yoga

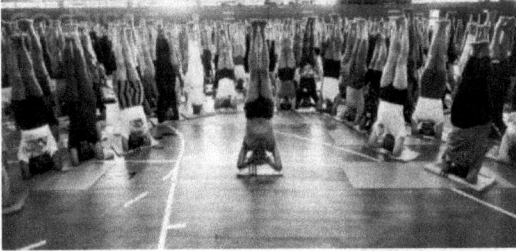

This is typically done by beginners and people who can only perform limited movements. The actions are subtle, but the focus is to perfect the proper alignment. There are certain poses that are done with props. This is done to make it easier for the practitioner to follow the steps.

When you are only starting with yoga, this gives you a peek as to the kinds of poses that you can do. It also makes you become aware of your physical strengths and weaknesses. It helps you in conquering the latter by improving your flexibility.

8. Jivamukti Yoga

This kind of yoga practice is both physically exhilarating and intellectually stimulating. It allows you to focus on your spiritual growth. It involves different sequences from various yoga practices, meditation and breathing techniques.

9. Kripalu Yoga

This kind of yoga can be extremely easy or quite tough. It forces you to observe the sensations of your body and mind. This way, you will understand how you are benefitting from a pose and how your life is being affected by the decisions that you make. This is achieved through meditation, relaxation, asana and pranayama. The goal is to awaken that natural life force that will help you cope with all areas of your life.

10. Kundalini Yoga

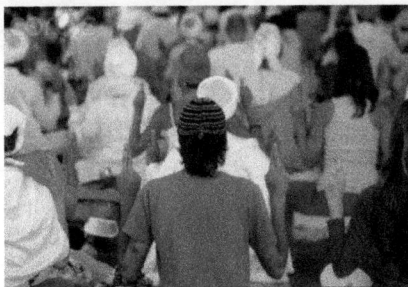

This aims to push your limits through extensive movements that are repeated within 90-minute duration of a class. It includes breathing exercises, mantras, mudras and mini-meditations. A typical class of this kind of yoga will usually start by performing a chant and singing by the end of the class. This is also referred to as the Yoga of Awareness, which is aimed towards the awakening of your kundalini energy. As you go through the process, you will have a thorough spiritual evaluation that will prompt your core to transform.

11. OM Yoga

The goal of this yoga is to process your strength and help you attain clarity and stability. It allows you to have more compassion with your life and how you live it. It is composed of Vinyasa sequences that are done at a moderate pace in alignment with the concepts of compassion and mindfulness.

12. ParaYoga

This combines dynamic practice with the Tantric philosophy. The classes are comprised of difficult asanas that allot lengthy time in practicing mudras, bandhas, pranayama and meditation. It teaches you how asana affects energy and how you can have a more refined prana and increased self-awareness.

13. Prana Flow Yoga

This is the kind of practice that is a fluid form of Vinsaya yoga, which teaches you how to connect with prana. It is both challenging and empowering. The class opens with Om, followed by near-continuous sequences that are creative and accompanied by music.

14. Purna Yoga

The classes are more focused in asanas with the incorporation of yogic philosophy and the alignment methods of Iyengar yoga. Quick meditations are done before and after each class, which is intended to connect the practitioners to the heart center. It hopes to teach you how to connect your body and mind to your spirit. It is comprised of four limbs, such as pranayama, asana, nutrition and lifestyle, and applied philosophy.

15. Sivananda Yoga

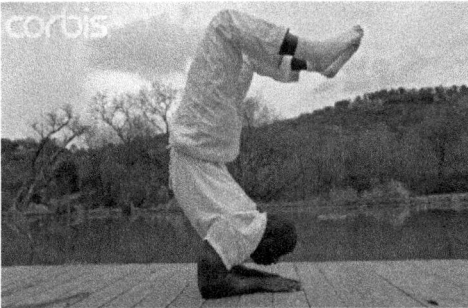

The practice is more spiritual than physical and is based on the teachings of Swami Sivananda. Each class typically lasts for 90 minutes. In this duration, you will perform

12 core poses, meditate, relax, practice pranayama and Sanskrit chanting. It aims to give you a higher consciousness. It focuses on the five fundamental yoga points, which are proper breathing, right exercise, Corpse pose, positive thinking and meditation, and vegetarianism or proper diet.

16. Svaroopa Yoga

Svaroopa means the bliss of your own Being. The classes involve a lot of floor work and hand movements. It opens and ends in Savasana or Corpse Pose. The goal is to release tension by creating a core opening that will remove everything that is stopping you from having an inner transformation.

17. TriYoga

The classes involve movements that are aimed to awaken your prana. It is composed of wavelike movements of the spine and coordinated breathing. You are expected to perform mudras, flowing asanas, dharana, pranayama and meditation.

18. Viniyoga

This is considered therapeutic and classes are designed based on the individual requirements of the practitioner. This will teach you to how to move the spine in accordance to your breathing. It also teaches you how to cultivate the positive and lessen the negative. This will lead you to the point of a discriminative awareness, which is important in order to achieve self-transformation.

These are only some of the yoga classes that you can look for. Decide which type best fits your need and requirements, and then search the areas near you for available classes or trainers. You can also study the yoga practices on your own, but make sure that you have the right materials and complete equipment before you begin.

CHAPTER 3: SIDDHASANA POSE

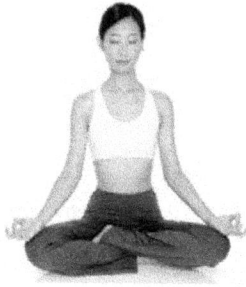

Some believe the best time to practice yoga exercises is the first thing in the morning before breakfast. Others believe the best time to practice yoga is in the evening, preparing the body for sleep; however, simply practicing when you are able will still allow you to reap the benefits of the practice.

Generally, yoga poses bring about a general sense of calm as it relieves stress, eliminates fatigue and refreshes the brain.

Muscle tissue stringency and stress could be rapidly alleviated by practicing yoga, and the asanas can also optimize blood circulation and enhance digestive function.

Many stress-related symptoms, such as fatigue, unbalanced emotions, inadequate quantity or quality of sleep, muscle tissue constrictions as well as anxiousness can be alleviated. Truly, the benefits of yoga are almost immeasurable.

Yoga takes a holistic approach regarding exercise, and its advantages encompass physical, mental and emotional health and wellness.

Regardless of age, yoga can significantly improve your quality of life. Yoga is gaining popularity and becoming one of the favored types of physical exercise with regard to its ability to affect a person's physical, mental and emotional health in one series of exercises.

According to research, yoga is viewed as a viable form of exercise because of the following physical benefits:

☐Boosting the body's flexibility.

☐Conditioning the movement of tendons, bones and ligaments.

☐ Internally massaging all the muscles, organs, tendons and ligaments of the body.

☐ Promoting optimal blood flow and bringing about 'detoxification.'

☐Promoting weight loss, toning the body, creating muscle definition and reducing overall body fat.

Yoga is recommended for people with stressful working conditions, those who suffer from headaches, those with back and joint pain, those with allergies and sensitivities, and those who suffer from asthma.

Yoga has been known to alleviate symptoms to such a degree that practitioners are able to forego or eliminate medications for physical ailments, anxiety and depression.

Doctors are beginning to recognize that yoga helps patients simply by enabling them to become their own internal expert and to increase their self-awareness.

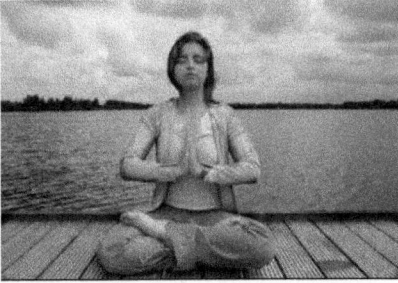

Yoga for Beauty – Proud posture, a graceful gait, a tuneful voice, glowing skin, an open and relaxed expression and appealing smile are ways that one's physical beauty may improve.

Through practicing the Yoga asanas on a regular basis, both men and women will achieve a strong body that will enhance their appearance and suppleness which gives them allure and elegance in every movement.

Having a glow from within affects one's personality, behavior and expression and often results in glowing skin, sparkling eyes and a radiant smile. Many world-famous celebrities practice yoga regularly and attribute it to helping them achieve success.

Following are some of the common ailments that can be healed by practicing yoga.

High Blood Pressure

Many people believe that practicing yoga might help lower blood pressure through inhaling and exhaling methods and lowering stress levels.

Regular physical exercise coupled with lifestyle changes can help reduce as well as handle hypertension. It is important to note that it does not necessarily do so in all situations.

Several yoga postures are designed to increase blood flow. Even the simplest posture, savasana, or dead body pose can assist with blood flow, particularly in the hands and feet.

Yoga encourages additional oxygen flow to your muscle tissue, which results in building and strengthening the muscle groups.

Turning and twisting postures are believed to permit oxygenated blood to flow to the organs in order to wring out toxins in the body.

Inversion postures, in which the head is upside down, encourage blood from your legs and pelvis to circulate and return to one's heart, where it can be pumped to the lung area to become oxygenated.

Inversion postures also send fresh, oxygenated blood to the brain resulting in improved mental clarity. Most appealing of all in regard to inversion postures is the age-rewind benefit. It is believed that the increased blood flow to the face discourages the face from wrinkling.

Research indicates that yoga increases production
of Hemoglobin and red-colored

bloodstream cells (RBC), which usually carry oxygen for the tissues.

It also encourages the blood to flow freely throughout the body preventing blood clots.

This may lead to a reduction in strokes and cerebral vascular accidents because blood clots are often the reason for these types of incidents.

If you begin a yoga practice, this not imply that you should discontinue using blood pressure medication if it is prescribed top you. You should never cease treatment without the expressed consent of your doctor.

Depression

Following just one single yoga class, practitioners documented diminishes in tension, fatigue, and frustration as well as an elevation of mood.

It is well documented that physical exercise including yoga contains a mood-elevating impact.

Immune System

It is believed that yoga contributes to strengthening the immune system. Those who practice yoga regularly report an overall reduction in the occurrence of illness as well as a reduction in the symptoms and duration of minor illnesses when they do occur.

Quality and Cognition of Life

Many people who suffer from serious and even terminal illnesses turn to yoga as an alternative treatment solution. Those who experience the often unpleasant side effects of treatment report enhancements in quality of life and as well as

an improvement in energy levels and a reduction in fatigue.

When muscles contract and stretch, bodily organs move internally resulting in a boost in water discharge and draining of the lymphatic system. This is the system that holds immune cells and boosts cellular functioning.

Diabetes

There is evidence that yoga might assist in lowering blood glucose levels. This has been known to reduce or eliminate the need for medication in certain practitioners who suffer from diabetes.

Yoga lowers cortisone levels resulting in increased production of the adrenal system and an increase in the performance of the immune system. Increased cortisone levels compromise the body's disease fighting capabilities and contribute to insulin resistance.

Higher cortisone amounts in the body lead to what scientists call "food-seeking behaviors" (which tend to manifest when you're upset, irritated, or even stressed).

In addition, increased cortisone levels are linked to an increase in abdominal fat which is linked to an increase in heart disease. Along with a healthy lifestyle plan that includes changes to the diet, yoga can enhance the body's ability to reduce abdominal fat and lower the risks associated with too much abdominal fat.

CHAPTER 4: THE FUNDAMENTALS OF YAMA

With Niyama peering inward, Yama counters by acting outward. One is contemplative, the other is proactive. The first is inward, the second is outward. It is balanced on multiple levels. Yama is a necessary and vital limb of the practice of Yoga because it unites what's inside with the outside. The study of the external is important to contrast the internal, but to also observe the internal within the grand scheme of things.

There is one more contrast that describes this limb. It is a list of what you should not do, versus the Niyama which is a list of things you should do. Just like the Niyama, the Yama has five areas that a person on the path of Yoga should avoid.

Non-Violence

The first element of Yama is to refrain from violence. Violence is a corruption of the mind that destroys the energy of life.

Life is not destroyed in the natural cycle of death and birth, it is destroyed when violence is driven by poor understanding and lack of self-control. Non-violence is called Ahimsa in Sanskrit. It is the core belief of all those who pursue the path of Yoga and it manifest as kindness to all living things. Yoga is about understanding, and it uses contemplation to get there. When needed, it uses rules as guidelines to be able to elevate the thought and spirit of the person. In this case of non-violence, it is not about the violence against the being and the effect it has on the being. This is not about sympathy. This is about what external violence does to the internal soul.

We live in a world where death and life are two sides of the same coin. Without life, there is no death, and without death, there can't be life. If you asked a lion to stop hunting its prey, you are sentencing that lion to death. So if non-violence and harm are bad, then how is that reconciled with the circle of life? The answer is simple. Killing is not violence when it is done in the natural course of things.

Non-violence in the mind is more important. When the frontier men hunt to put food on the table, there is no violence to speak of. But when a man hunts for sport and finds pleasure in the death of another the soul of the man is altered. When man defends his own life when attacked and injures his assailant, that is not violence, but protection.

Truth

The next Yama is the truth, or Satya, in Sanskrit. Satya is not about telling the truth, it is beyond that. Satya is about seeking the truth and putting one's self on the path to recognize the truth. To see the truth requires contemplation and reflection. It requires one's mindset to be different from those who traffic in lies and are blind to the truth. It takes a special kind of mind to deal in falsehoods. A mind that deals in falsehoods can never see the truth of the Universe even if it is right in front of them. Shakespeare says, in Hamlet, "to thine own self be true."

To seek the truth in Yoga is a simple affair. If you make it a practice to see the truth, then you will be able to see things as they are. Understanding the truth and seeing this as they allow you to understand this Universe instead of being blinded by the bright lights that distract. The lack of peace in a person and the corresponding stresses that develop are frequently because we have failed to see the truth. No one is lying to the person who cannot see the truth for himself. Even if another person speaks falsely, if you are not blind, you will be able to see through them. What happens when you do not know what the truth looks like?

Yoga is about seeing things as they are and that is more so in this element of Yama. Once again it is about looking outside and seeing the truth for yourself. All the while, as you are looking for the external truth, you are clearing your lenses of the limitations that you have inadvertently accumulated. The path to Yoga removes those blinders and allows you to see things for what they are.

Covetousness

To be covetous is to desire what another person possesses. In this world of social media shares, likes, and influencers, many have become the exact opposite of that. To understand what one thinks of a product is one thing; to want what someone else has, is quite another.

Being covetous for things shields you from your desires. We underestimate our ability to know what is good and what is not good in our own life. The subconscious faculties that conjure desire and aversion, do so to propel us in certain directions. They have aggregated our whole being and determined our most effective path. If they find that something is deficient in that journey, it shows up as a desire. That desire is born from within. Imagine cooking a dish, and just before applying the final touches, one samples it. That sample reveals that it is deficient in flavor – specifically salt. The solution is simple, one would then reach for the salt and add the necessary sprinkles. Not more, not less. More would signify greed. Less would render the dish less than perfect for one's taste. There is also another dimension to that. Hypothetically, if another was preparing the same dish, and they needed to add sugar to their final product, would following them at this juncture, yield positive results for you? No.

Being covetous of someone's actions, possessions, or lifestyle, will negatively impact what we have to offer. It is not wrong to desire anything when that desire comes from deep within us. But when that desire is driven by an external source, it becomes incompatible with who we are, where we are at that time. In Yoga, this is called Asteya.

Self-Restraint

While this feature may seem like it is about an internal process and should be listed in the Niyama versus here, in the Yama, self-restraint is about external stimulus affecting an internal response. During early development, creatures were reactive. The development of the brain was in response to something external. In many ways, our evolution is a response to external factors. But those are organic, and well-balanced advances.

Self-restraint is about reactions to primal desires created in areas that exceed what we are originally designed to do. Take obesity for instance. When it is not a genetic issue, obesity is more about the inability to control the consumption of food. There is no self-restraint in this case. The result is the imbalance of desires and the destruction of the mind.

This self-restraint requirement within Yama is specifically directed toward the lack of restraint in sexual desire. Yoga does not need one to be celibate within the confines of one's relationship. Yoga is not talking about the act, but rather, the runaway desire that leads to the act. Desires for sex beyond what it is designed to do renders the person a slave to the desire and distracted from the other areas of one's life. It is hard to recognize the truth that is all around us when we are constantly thinking of a biological desire like sex or food.

In Yoga, this is called Brahmacharya and it is an important element in one's spiritual and mental development. The prevalence of sexual desire says two things about us. The first is that we are swayed by the programming of the primal mind. The second is that we are distracted by something external.

The inability to control the desire is the focal point, not the ability to have the desire. The difference between the two that needs attention is not that the response is triggered, but that the desire can't be controlled.

Non-Possessive

In Sanskrit, it is called Aparigraha. It is the ability to not want to own or rather, the understanding that we are not here to own. From Yoga's perspective, imagine the Universe to be a sheet of fabric. Each weave and each part of the cloth is a phenomenon of its own – the planets, the celestial bodies, the elements, and even more complex occurrences, like life, which is a combination of the elements and forces. We are all part of the same fabric. Seeking to possess something that is also part of that cloth, would be like our left hand trying to possess the right. It is not natural. We cannot possess what we are already a part of.

The only thing we can own is the responsibility to serve as part of that cloth, not to own it. The desire to own it is misplaced and can cause confusion and disappointment. Possessions cloud the mind and blind the eye. It is difficult to understand or recognize the truth when one is blind.

CHAPTER 5: YOGA POSTURES FOR WEIGHT LOSS

Weight loss is an integral component of yoga. Many people practice yoga to have control of their body and ultimately shed weight and get a perfect and lean figure. Weight loss through yoga isn't a one-week affair and takes several months of training and regular yoga. You will have to perfect a few of the yoga poses to lose weight.

Here are few of the best postures in yoga practice for weight loss:

Warrior Pose

For this pose, stand upright with your legs far apart. Raise your hands above your head and stretch them as much as possible. Clasp your hands together to make a Namaste gesture and turn yourself to the right. Bend your right knee a little while trying to stretch your abdominal muscles as much as possible. Repeat the procedure on the left side. This is beneficial as it tightens your muscles and reduces fat deposited in the legs giving you an impressive body built.

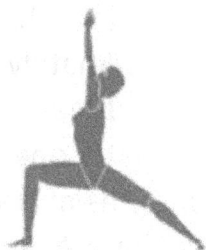

Warrior Pose II

This yoga pose is very similar to the previous Warrior pose I; however, it focuses on the abdominal muscles. It has the same effect on the tummy and legs, yet it is done in a unique way. The hands do not make a Namaste gesture but are stretched out on both the sides while the leg is bent. This pose ensures that the abdominal muscles are stretched which makes it very effective for fat elimination.

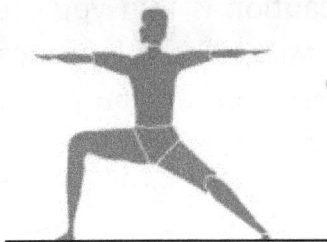

Chair Pose

This pose requires a lot of stamina. Start by keeping your feet together, and inhale as you raise your hands above head level. Stretch your hands up and bend your knees slightly, make sure you keep inhaling while bending. Now the difficult part; hold this position for at least 60 seconds. It may seem difficult in the beginning to remain in this position, so practice it as much as you can and stand back up when you feel uncomfortable or pressured. For starters, you can begin by practicing it 10 times every day and increase the time as well as the frequency after every 3 days.

I point of caution is that you are likely to experience pain in your legs for the initial couple of days but as you practice it, the pain eases out. This pose is very effective for helping you have toned thighs, for getting rid of tummy fat as well as enhances your flexibility.

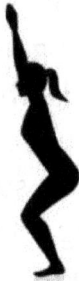

Boat Pose

For this posture, sit down on your yoga mat and stretch your legs out. Your knees should be pulled up, thighs should be kept tight, and toes pointed out. Now gradually raise your feet off the ground and set them at a 45-degree angle. Keep inhaling as you raise your feet and try not to bend your knees. Keep your spine erect to make sure your body forms a V shape and then raise your arms up to the shoulder. This pose will improve your stamina and cut down on your tummy fat. It will also increase your lower and upper body strength.

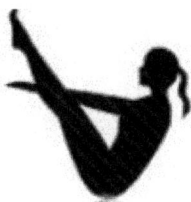

Bridge Pose

Lie down on your back and bend your knees, ensuring that your feet are firmly on the ground. Put your hands on the ground and keep them straight. Now raise your hips from the ground and try to balance your body only using your hands and feet.

This pose will improve your muscle strength and efficiency. You can also experiment by adding variations to this pose. Try to lift one leg in the air for longer periods and then do the same with your

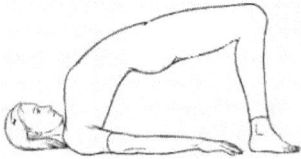

other leg.

Cobbler's pose

The Yoga cobbler's pose is one of the simplest of all yoga poses. All you need to do is sit down with your spine erect. Your knees should be bent and the soles of your feet facing each other. Press your soles together and hold this pose for at least a minute.

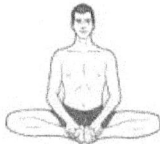

Locust Pose

For the Yoga Locust pose, lie face down while your palms face the ground. Inhale a burst of fresh air while lifting up your legs without bending your knees. The upper side of your stomach and hands should also be lifted to stretch your abdominal muscles. This way, you can balance yourself by the tummy. This pose helps you to minimize the fat zones near the hips and expand the ability of your leg muscles.

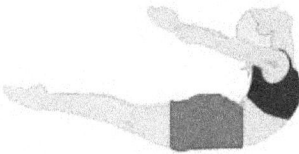

Camel Pose

Sit on your feet with your knees and calves very close. You will have to place a soft cloth under to prevent pain. After doing so, come onto your knees and place your hands on your hips while stretching out the torso. Hold your heels gradually one after the other and try to bend backward to expand your chest and tummy.

You are likely to feel the weight of your body in your arms. This pose is very beneficial in reducing accumulated fat in almost all the areas of the body.

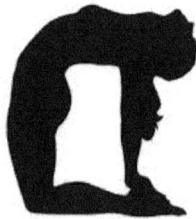

By practicing the yoga postures mentioned above, you will be able to effectively and efficiently stretch your muscles especially around legs, abdomen, hands, waist and hips. This will burn most of your fats and even give you a healthier, nicely shaped body. Moreover, conditions like constipation, stress and hypersensitivity are significantly reduced when you practice most of these poses.

Now that we have looked as some amazing poses to help you lose weight, let us look at other poses that are very effective for stress relief.

CHAPTER 6: HOW BREATHING AFFECTS THE BODY

As you practice yoga, nothing is as important as breathing deeply and holding your breath for as long as possible. This is important because holding your breath as you practice whichever asana will ensure you reap the benefits of that specific asana.

Deep/abdominal breathing technique, also called **diaphragmatic breathing,** involves the diaphragm, an important large muscle located between your abdomen and your chest.

When your diaphragm contracts, it moves downward, a movement that leads to the expansion of the abdomen. This process mounts a negative pressure on your chest and forces air into your lungs. This negative pressure helps pull blood into your chest. It also enhances the flow of lymph, known to be rich in immune cells. This causes relaxation of your nervous system and reversal of the stimulation of your parasympathetic nervous system.

Deep breathing is very vital to your overall health and wellbeing. When you engage in yoga and practice deep breathing, you induce a series of physical responses that reverse the changes brought about by stressful, depressive situations. This is how deep/abdominal breathing improves immunity, prevents lung and tissue infections, and induces the relaxation response that leads to less tension and improved general wellbeing.

The calming and reversing effect brought about by deep breathing during yoga happens through the reduction of your heart rate, the tension in your muscles, and by calming your nerves. Since breathing is so important to enjoying the benefits of yoga, it is very important that you learn good breathing techniques. The basics of every deep breathing exercise are to inhale deeply through your nostrils while drawing deeply from your diaphragm/abdomen.

Now that we have established the importance of deep breathing during yoga, let us discuss how to breathe deeply so you can derive the benefits of yoga:

How to Practice Deep/Abdominal Breathing

This type of breathing requires some level of training and mastery before you can get it right. You can follow the steps below to get the best from your deep breathing during yoga exercises:

Keep one hand placed on your chest and one on your abdomen. As you inhale through your nostril, the hand on the abdomen ought to rise higher than the one on your chest. This way, you can be sure you are pulling air into the base of your lungs.

As you inhale through your nostrils, visualize the air in the room going into your airways and count from 1-7 while you hold your breath.

Count from 1-8 as you exhale through your mouth. Gently contract your abdominal muscles to ensure any remaining air evacuates your lungs.

You can regulate your breath by taking an average of 6 breaths every minute. Repeat this deep/abdominal breathing technique for about 5 times before switching to a different yoga pose.

Having mastered the act of deep/abdominal breathing, let us now look at how, by using different yoga poses, you can achieve different ends such as boosting immunity, building stamina, and fighting stress and anxiety.

Before we do that, however, let us lay some ground rules for your yoga practice.

Yoga Practice for Beginners: General Guidelines

As a beginner, you need to learn and pay attention to a few yoga rules/guidelines especially because adhering to these guidelines will see you enjoy the best of yoga benefits.

Here are some of the most important yoga rules/guidelines you must adhere to as a beginner:

NOTE: Always begin by meditating briefly and setting an intention for your yoga practice

Your yoga practice should always start with a brief meditation session coupled with setting an intention for the yoga exercise. A brief mindful meditation session before yoga is important because it helps you achieve the level of awareness you need to make the best of your yoga exercise.

Your brief meditation should center on mindful breathing focusing on the duration and sensation of your breaths and probably the number of breaths you take per minute. You can try the deep breathing exercise discussed above to help build your awareness on the present before you start practicing any yoga pose.

Also, you can practice mindfulness by being aware of the feelings on various parts of your body as you start engaging in yoga, during a session and after a session. For instance, feel the tension on your muscles, the feel of air touching your skin, the posture you've taken, the feel on your body (from the toes to the top of your head etc.).

When it comes to setting intention for your yoga practice, your intention can be anything ranging from your need to achieve inner peace, to gaining an attitude of gratitude, to building self-discipline, to building self-confidence, to beating mental disorders such as anxiety, depression, stress, fear, etc.

1: Go For Yoga Asanas You Are Most Comfortable With

Your body type and weight play largely determine which yoga poses work for you and which ones you find complicated. Experimenting with different poses depending on the goal of your yoga practice will help you choose the poses most suitable for your body type/weight and the purpose for which you are embracing yoga.

2: Go For Poses Done On the Floor

Irrespective of your energy levels and stamina, if you are just getting started on yoga, you will succeed more if you go for yoga poses you can do while lying on the floor or on your yoga mat than when you choose difficult poses that require you stand for a period.

Yoga poses done on the floor—poses such as the fish pose, corpse pose, or baby pose—do not require much strength or balance.

3: Regulate the Intensity of Your Yoga Practices

How challenging and vigorous your yoga practice is will depend on what you can handle as a beginner. It is best to begin with slow and simple steps/poses and ensure you understand postures and alignments before going for more challenging ones.

4: Practice Duration

The length and duration of your yoga practice will also depend on your yoga goals, your schedule, and ability. However, it is more beneficial to engage in frequent yoga practices for short periods than it is to engage in yoga practices that last extended periods occasionally.

To get the best from your yoga practices, commit to 10-20 minutes per period at least 2-8 times per week.

5: Location

Like your mindful meditation exercise, your yoga practices require solitude and quietness. If you choose to practice at home, make sure you time your sessions to fall into periods when the house is quiet. The early morning hours are ideal for practicing yoga at home. Alternatively, you can practice your yoga exercises in yoga studios near you, gardens, etc.

6: Yoga Clothes

When it comes to yoga clothing, choose clothing that will not restrict your movements as you cycle through the various asanas. The best clothing for yoga is loose comfortable clothes or body-fitted tops and pants.

7: Foods and Drinks

Eating or drinking a few minutes to your yoga practice is not advisable. The best practice is to eat about 3 hours before your yoga sessions and drink very small amounts of any liquids before engaging in your yoga practice. You must try not to drink anything all through the duration of your yoga practice.

Before you get started, it is important that you are aware of some contraindications regarding yoga to ensure you are fit for the practice.

Contraindications

Every yoga posture and technique comes with its unique contraindications; however, there are general don'ts when it comes to yoga practices. The following conditions require special care and your doctor's opinion before you engage in any yoga pose.

Pregnancy

Menstruation

Neck injuries

Knee injuries

Back injuries

Shoulder injuries

High blood pressure

Now that we have looked at the various yoga benefits, the importance of mindful deep breathing, and the key guidelines you should follow as you practice yoga, let us get to the actual practice: the asanas you should practice to experience the benefits we discussed earlier:

CHAPTER 7: GREAT YOGA POSES

Asana or body position is closely associated with Yoga. Asana or Yoga poses are marked as the mastery of sitting still. Yoga is a form of physical exercise but its modern day version inculcates various transformations. Asana maintain the vitality and flexibility of the practitioners and thus, promotes over-all wellness. Yoga is also popular as Alternative Medicine in West, while it is believed to be spiritual self-mastery meditation skill, in the East. There is a group of classic 84 asanas in Yoga preached by Lord Shiva, mentioned in the ancient and classic text of yoga. The explanation of these Yoga Asanas, is texted in:

Patanjali's Yoga Sutra

Hatha Yoga Samhita

Goksha Samhita

Hatha Ratnavali

Gheranda Samhita

A few benefits of Asana or Yoga poses and postures are:

Enhances Strengthen

Improves Flexibility

Promotes Balance and Equilibrium

Improves Sleep Disturbances

Prevents Diabetes Complications

Heals Lower Back Pain and Problems

Eradicates Anxiety and Stress

Fruitful for Chronic Pulmonary Disease (COPD)

Decreases Labor Pain

Promotes Fertility in Men and Women

Cures Hypertension

Remedy for Diabetes Management

Prevents Ageing

Effective for Elderly

Natrajasana (Dancing Shiva)

This pose stretches the abdominal, neck muscles, and tones the hips. It works wonders and improves the digestion and makes the spine, supple.

Directions:

Begin by lying down on the floor. Bend your right knee and place right foot on the outside of the left knee. Stretch both the arms to the sides at shoulder length.

Breathe the air in. While exhaling, twist the torso to the left side and head to the alternate side right. Look over the right shoulder.

Press the right thigh towards the floor, by keeping the shoulders on the ground. You can incorporate your left hand to your thigh further down.

Hold the pose and take long deep breaths.

Relax the body through exhale.

Repeat the activity by following the same procedure on the other side.

Vajrasana (Thunderbolt Pose)

Vajra means diamond shape and asana means posture and hence, it's called Vajraasana. During the pranayams, it is advisable to sit in Vajrasana (Adamantine Pose).The pose is essential in enhancing the blood circulation to body and improving the digestive system. It is a perfect pose, to ease digestion. It relives, bloating, gas and flatulence. This pose strengthens the muscles of thigh and legs. It reduces rheumatic disease by making the ankle and knee joints flexible. It erects the spine and is practiced before pranayama.

Directions:

Keep the hips on the heels by folding the legs inwards. Toes must point out behind and big toes must touch each other.

Sit on the fit constructed by the parted heels.

Hold the pose for some time and take deep and long breaths.

Breathe out and relax. Straighten your legs after completing a cycle.

Trikonasana (Triangle Pose)

This yoga pose strengthens the knees, ankles, chest, arms and legs. It effectively stretches the groins, hips, hamstrings, shoulders, chest and spine. It is best known to enhance the physical and mental equilibrium. It helps improve the digestion process. This yoga posture reduces back pain, sciatica, anxiety and stress.

Directions:

Stand straight. Separate the two feet wide apart comfortably.

Turn your right root out (90 degrees) and left foot in (15 degrees).

Align the center of right heel with the center of arch of left foot.

Balance the body weight equally on both feet by pressing them towards the ground.

Inhale deep breaths and as you exhale out, bend your body to the right, downward from the hips, by keeping the waist straight. Allow your left hand to be lifted in the air while your right hand should come down towards the ground. Keep both the arms in a straight line.

Relax your right hand on your ankle, shin or on the floor outside your right foot, whatever is feasible, without disturbing the sides of the waist. Stretch your left arm towards the ceiling, in line with your shoulders. Keep the head neutral or turn it to the left side, with eyes gazing softly at the left palm.

Ensure that your body is bent sideways and not forward or backward. The chest and pelvis must be wide open.

Stretch to your maximum potential and be in a steady state. Continue inhaling and exhaling and constantly relax the body.

As you inhale, bring your arms down to your respective sides and straighten out your feet.

Repeat the same procedure on other side as well.

Shavasana (Corpse Pose)

This pose is meant to relax and help the body, to rest. This posture is excellent in bringing, meditative deep state of rest, which aids the body to repair the cells and tissues, by releasing stress. It helps the practitioner to reach a deeper level of mind. The pose fosters rejuvenation and is critical pose, to end any yoga session. It reduces anxiety, insomnia and blood pressure. It even diminishes the Vata Dosha (imbalance of the air element).

Directions:

Begin by lying flat on the ground, without incorporating cushions and props. If it is absolutely necessary, use a small cushion, to rest the head. Close both your eyes.

Relax your feet and knees by keeping the legs comfortably apart with topes facing the sides.

Locate your arms alongside, yet a little spaced apart, from the body. Rest your palms open by facing them downwards.

Relax your whole body by taking the attention to your different parts of your body by focusing one by one.

Commence by bringing the awareness to the right foot and move to the right knee (after completing one leg, concentrate on the other leg) and gradually move upwards by relaxing and calming your all body parts.

Breathe gently, deeply and slowly and allow yourself to relax at every breath inhaled or exhaled. The inhaled breath energizes the body while the exhaled one relaxes the cells of the body. Avoid sleeping but forgo all the stress, emergencies and hurry. Surrender yourself completely to your breaths.

Repeat the procedure and after a short duration you would feel relaxed and rejuvenated. Keep your eyes close and gradually roll onto your right side. Stay in the same position for some quality time. Now, with the support of your right hand, gently leave the position and sit up. Remain in Sukhsana (Easy pose) for a few minutes.

Stay in the position with your eyes closed and take a few deep breaths and slowly become conscious of your environment. Restore yourself and open your closed eyes to enlightenment.

Ardha Chakrasana (Standing Forward Bend)

It is a best pose for stretching the front upper torso. Ardha Chakrasana is popular as it tones up the arms and shoulders

Directions:

Stand straight with feet held together and arms along-side the body.

Maintain the balance of your weight on both the feet,

Inhale while extending your arms over the head, while palms still facing downwards.

Exhale and gently bend backwards, pushing the pelvis forward while keeping the arms in the line with elbows and ears. Keep the knees straight with head held up and lift your chest towards the ceiling.

Hold the pose and continue to breathe in and out.

Breathe out and bring the arms down and relax the body.

Hanumanasana (Monkey Pose)

This yoga posture strengthens and stretchers the muscles in thigh, groin region and hamstrings. Hanumansana stimulates the lower and upper abdominal organs and hence improves their functioning. This posture makes the high more flexible.

Directions:

Commence by kneeling on the floor with knees distanced a little wide apart. Place your right foot forward and uplift your inner sole at such a height so as outer heel only touches the floor.

As you breathe out bend your torso forward and bring your fingertips to touch the ground.

Gradually move your left knee backwards until the knee and the front of the touch completely touch the ground. Simultaneously slide your right leg forward until and unless it touches the floor.

Retain a same position by sliding tour left foot backward and right foot forward.

The toes should be the opposite direction as the right foot should point towards the sky while the left foot should be placed touching the ground.

Raise you're both arms upwards and join both the palms. Stretch your arms gradually and arch your back behind a little.

Maintain this position for a couple of minutes before bringing your arms back to the normal position.

To withdraw the posture; shift the entire weight of the body on the respective hands by pressing them slowly towards the ground. Gradually slide your right and left feet back to the initial position before repeating the cycle with the left leg in the front and right leg behind.

Marjari Asana (Cat Stretch)

Marjari asana or the cat pose restores the flexibility of the spine. It is very effective in strengthening the shoulders and the wrists. It is excellent for digestive system as it improves digestion, by massaging the digestive systems. It is ideal for toning the abdomen. Cat pose improves blood circulation and therefore, supplies more oxygen to the body. It works wonder by relieving the stress and relaxes the mind.

Directions:

Come on to all fours, by sitting on your knees. Gain a position that is familiar to a table with your back as a table top and your hand and feet forming the legs of the table.

Rest your arms perpendicular to the floor and keep your hands directly under the shoulders and stay them flat on the ground. Your knees should be placed at hip-width apart.

Repaet this by a countermovement, As you breathe out, raise your chin and tilt your head back, while pushing the navel downwards and uplift you tailbone. Compress your buttocks.

Retain this poses for a few seconds before attaining the initial table like position.

Continue six to seven cycles, before withdrawing the posture.

Chapter 8: Yoga For Stress Relief

One of the main benefits of yoga is stress relief. By focusing on your mind and body, you gain a sense of peace and restfulness that is helpful to reduce the amount of stress that you feel in your mind. It doesn't make the problems go away, but it can help you to stay calm and focused in order to solve life's problems. No one likes to feel stressed out.

While some poses are good for weight loss, others are more effective for stress relief. In this chapter, we're going to take a look at the poses that are good for stress relief when performed on a regular basis. If you need to relieve some stress in your life, then try some of these poses to try and calm your mind.

Seal Pose

The seal pose is designed to help you bring your mental, physical and emotional issues together and get centered. This pose consists of putting your palms together over your chest near your heart. The physical motion helps you to be physically centered. By using this pose with meditation, you can help center your mind and emotions as well. While holding this pose, focus on your breathing and clearing your mind. Take slow breaths and feel the positive energy in your body. Do this for as long as you still feel stressed.

The seal pose is a great pose to perform in the spur of the moment. When you're feeling overwhelmed, just take a moment and focus on becoming more centered and letting the stress out.

Easy Pose

This pose is the pose most people think about when thinking about yoga. In this pose, you sit on the floor, cross-legged. Place your hands palm up on your knees and sit up straight with your shoulders back. While concentrating on your breathing or meditating on something that calms you, you sit with your hand on your knees and just focus. This helps you become more grounded.

The Cat Pose

This pose consists of being on your hands and knees with your spine arched back.This helps your inner systems to flow more freely and helping you to feel like your energy is flowing and in sync.While doing this pose, make sure that you're concentrating on your breathing. Hold this pose and allow your body to feel the stretch.

These are just a few of the poses that can help you relieve stress. Stress relief poses can be performed almost anywhere whenever you need to do them. If you're having a stressful day at work, take some time and do the seal pose or the easy pose. By taking a few minutes to get yourself centered and grounded, you will be able to push away the stress and handle the situations as they come.

Yoga helps you become balanced not only physically, but also mentally. Finding a yoga pose that will help you release your stress at its onset will help you to find peace and harmony in difficult situations. Even if you don't have time for a full workout, find a pose that will help center you so that you can keep going with whatever tasks are at hand. You will be glad you did. You will feel better and less stressed out by many circumstances that affect your daily life.

Hatha Yoga

When most Western people think of yoga, they are typically thinking of **Hatha** yoga and in particular it's postures, or **asanas** as they are known in Sanskrit.

There are hundreds of different asanas, which can be arranged in thousands of different routines. The following routine is aimed at beginners and provides a gentle but exhaustive full body routine.

Mountain Pose

One of the most basic yoga poses, is the **Mountain Pose.** Stand with your body stretched outright, feet against each other and weight rested evenly on both soles.

Inhale slowly. As you inhale raise your arms directly above your head, keeping your palm shoulder length apart, facing another. Extend your back and reach towards the sky. Exhale slowly as you release the posture.

Downward Dog

The downward dog is also a staple of most yoga routines. This simple movement strengthens the glutes, abs and thighs. Start by resting on all fours, with your back horizontal as your knees and palms flat against the floor. Gradually move your hands several spaces forward and stretch out your fingers. Your back should have a mild diagonal slant against the floor.

Curl your toes inwards and raise your hips towards the sky, forming an upside down V shape with your body. Keep your head align with your spine. Hold this position whilst you slowly inhale and exhale three times.

Warrior Pose

Another simple asana, the warrior position starts in a standing position, with the legs 4 feet apart. Keep the foot in front of your body facing directly forward, whilst twist your back foot slightly horizontally.

Raise your palms to your hips, but rest your shoulder muscles. Raise your arms to shoulder height, forming a straight line from palm to palm.

Balance more weight on your forward facing foot until your knee is above your ankle. Hold this position for 1 minute, inhaling and exhaling calmly whilst you do so. Repeat this asana with the alternate foot forward.

Tree Pose

Stand upright. Raise one foot and rest its sole on the opposing thigh, balancing your weight on the remaining foot. Bring your palms together in front on your ribs, as if you were praying. As you gently inhale, raise your arms above your shoulders vertically, with your palms facing each other. Hold this position for 30 seconds. As you exhale, release the position. Repeat this asana with your weight resting on the opposite foot.

Forward Bend

Stand upright with your feet touching each other and your weight evenly distributed. Slowly, as you exhale, push your chin into your chest and bend at the hips, bringing your upper half the body towards the floor. Reach to touch the floor with your fingers and your palms (if you can without pain). Hold this pose for 15 seconds, removing your fingers from the floor and returning to an upright position as you exhale.

Bridge Pose

Lay down on the yoga mat, with your knees bent above your ankles and the soles of your feet touching the floor. Place your palms against the floor behind your head. Push upwards from your palms whilst raising your hips. Hold this pose for 15-30 seconds, releasing during an exhalation.

High Lunge

Kneel on the yoga mat, with your weight balanced on your palms and knees. Your shoulders should be above your palms and your hips should be above your knees.

As you breathe out, position your left leg between your two palms, ensuring that the knee is still above the ankle. You may need to raise your back and bring your knee close to your collarbone to accomplish this.

Lift your torso upwards and raise your arms towards the sky, with the palms facing towards each other. Retain this posture for 15-30 seconds. During an exhalation, revert the movement so that you are once more resting on the floor with your weight balanced on your knees and palms.

Repeat the posture, moving the alternate leg forward.

Triangle Pose

Stand upright, with your legs roughly 3ft apart. Raise your arms so that they are horizontal align with your shoulders and your palms point towards the floor. Twist your right foot so that it points in front of you and twist your left foot so that it points towards the side. Move to reach the floor with your right hand, whilst simultaneously lifting your left hand towards the ceiling. Hold this posture for a moment, then revert back to an upright standing position as you next exhale.

Repeat this posture with the alternate foot facing forward.

Seated Twist

Sit on the yoga mat, with both your legs pointing forward. Raise your left leg over the right leg, placing the sole of the left foot against your right knee. Meanwhile move your left palm so that it rests on your right knee, whilst moving your right palm behind your back, to balance your weight and act as a support. Twist your body away from your left leg. Retain this position for 15-30 seconds, releasing this position as you exhale.

Repeat this posture moving the right leg over the left leg and using your left palm to support your weight.

Cobra Pose

Lay on the yoga mat, with your face to the floor. Place your palms to the side of your shoulders, so that your thumb just rests slightly under your shoulder. Push up from your palms, lifting your torso, tensing your glutes and pushing your hips to the ground. Hold this position for 30 seconds before releasing as you exhale. Repeat twice more.

Crow Pose

Kneel on the yoga mat, with your palms in front of your body and resting on the floor. Budge your knees up to your palms, so that your legs are right against your arms. Shift your weight forward, resting your entire weight on your palms and lifting your lower body into the air. Rest your knees against your arms for support. Tense your abs and attempt to hold this position for 10-15 seconds.

Hare Pose

Start in a kneeling position, with your bottom touching the floor and your feet by the side of your glutes with your body upright. Your palms should be resting on your thighs. Move your palms forward extending your back and lowering your head to the floor. Hold this pose for 15 seconds, releasing the pose during an exhalation.

Cat Pose

Kneel on the yoga mat, with your weight balanced on your palms and knees. Your shoulders should be above your palms and your hips should be above your knees. Raise your chin upwards whilst pushing your back downwards.

Hold this posture for a short moment. Reverse the position by lowering your chin in line with your arms whilst raising and arching your back. Hold this position for a short moment. Repeat this transformation 2-3 times.

Easy Plow Pose

Lay down on the yoga mat with your palms facing floor-down, resting by your hips. Bend your knees so that the sole of your feet is raised above the ground, but the tips of your toes touch the ground. Lift your legs and bend your torso on itself, being your legs over your head until your toes touch the floor behind you. Lock your hands together in front of your body. Finally lower your legs and bend your knees, so that your knees rest upon your forehead and your toes point towards the ceiling. Hold this posture for 15 seconds, releasing upon an exhalation.

Pigeon Pose

Kneel on the yoga mat, with your weight balanced on your palms and knees. Your shoulders should be above your palms and your hips should be above your knees.

Push up from your toes then bring your right leg forward and bend it around the front of your body so that the roof of your right foot touches the left palm.

 Meanwhile lower the left leg so that the roof of the left foot touches the floor. Bring your palms forward, lowering your head and torso over your right leg. Ensure your elbows are touching the floor. Hold this position for 15 seconds, releasing the posture during an exhalation. Repeat this posture with the alternate leg forward.

Bound Angle Pose

Sit with your legs facing forward and your palms on your thighs. Bend your knees, bringing the soles of your feet together by your groin. Place your hands over your feet. Hold this pose for 15-30 seconds, releasing the posture as you exhale.

Knee Press

Lay down on the floor. Raise your legs over your torso, bending your knees, pressing your thighs to your stomach. Bring your arms over your knees, locking them into place. Hold this posture for 15-30 seconds, releasing as you exhale.

Bow Pose

Lie on the floor face down, ensuring your legs are hips width apart. Bend your knees over your thighs. Bring your arms behind your body and grab your ankles with your palms. Lift your thighs and upper body together, pulling with your arms as you do so. Keep your head forward and your feet pointing towards the ceiling.

Garland Pose

Stand upright, with your feet just a little more than shoulder width apart. Bend your knees, squatting and bringing your buttocks to below knee level. Brace yourself by pushing your elbows in your thighs and bringing your palms together by your chest. Hold this pose for up to 15 seconds, releasing during an exhalation.

Upward Extended Feet

Lie down on the yoga mat, with your palms face down by your sides. Bend your knees, bringing your feet closer to your buttocks and raising your legs into the air. Hold this posture for 15 seconds, releasing your posture as you exhale.

Chair Pose

Stand upright, with your legs together. Raise your arms straight above your head, bringing your palms within 1-2 inches of each other. Bend your knees as much as you are possible. Slightly bend your back forwards, keeping your arms in the air. Hold this posture for 15 seconds, releasing during an exhalation.

Half-boat pose

Sit on the yoga mat with your legs straight out in front of you. Bend your knees and place your hands behind your back for support, as you tilt your back slightly backwards. Lift your legs in a half-bent way, so that your feet and shins point forward. Raise your arms to be parallel to your shins, palms facing inward, but not touching your legs. Hold this posture for 15 seconds, before releasing it during an exhalation.

Child Pose

Sit in a kneeling position, with your buttocks resting on your feet. Bend your torso forward, bringing your forehead all the way to the ground. Move your arms behind your body, with your palms touching your feet. Hold this posture for 15 seconds before releasing the pose during an exhalation.

Locust Pose

Lie face-down to the floor. Press your chin to the yoga mat. Press your arms under your hips, keeping your palms extended. Raise both your back legs in the air, ensuring you support the movement with the muscles in your back. Hold this posture for 15 seconds, making sure that you do not hold your breath whilst you do so.

One-arm advanced left bend

Stand upright, with your feet roughly shoulder width apart. Raise your right arm in the air and bend your torso to the left, whilst looking upwards at your arm in the air. Hold this posture for 15-30 seconds, before repeating it using the left arm and bending to the right.

Staff Pose

Kneel on the yoga mat, with your weight balanced on your palms and knees. Your shoulders should be above your palms and your hips should be above your knees. Bend you knees slightly and raise your feet so you are balancing on your toes. Descend your torso downwards, keeping your weight on your palms and your torso above the ground. Hold this posture for 15-30 seconds, releasing the pose during an exhalation.

Other Poses

These two following poses do not challenge the muscles, but they are still useful to maintain for relaxation and meditation purposes.

Corpse Pose

Lie on your back. Shift your back upwards on the mat, straightening and extending your spine. Meanwhile, straighten your legs, keeping your toes pointed upwards. Your arms should rest by your side, with your palms resting toward the ceiling. Your body should be extended and slightly stretched, but relaxed. This is a great posture to relax, meditate and breathe and be calm; use it whenever you need to unwind.

Perfect Pose

Sit on the floor with your legs facing forward. Bend your right leg, bring the sole of your foot against your buttocks. Bend your left leg and rest it over your right leg, with the sole of the left foot touching the right thigh. Place your hands on your knees, bringing your index finger and thumb together. Shuffle slightly to ensure you weight is evenly rested between your legs. Keep your back straight, but relax your shoulders and core. This is a good posture to meditate to mediate and experiment with the breathing.

Chapter 10: Tips For Yoga Beginners

Yoga has been proven to have many different health benefits, both psychological and physiological.It is an ancient practice, but it has very practical applications in this new day and age.Before you get started with yoga you might want to ask yourself a few questions.These are meant to get your mind into the right mindset before you begin. Why do I want to start yoga? Are my goals realistic? Do I have any physical limitations that might put me at greater risk of injury than other people? Do I have clear and definable goals? Am I ready to commit to a program? Will my family and friends support me, and if they don't, will I be able to handle it?

When looking for a yoga instructor, you might want to visit a few of their classes first to get a feel for the style of the individual. Some people claim to be yoga instructors but actually know very little about it. So that is an obvious concern.You may also have to deal with instructors who are angry or violent.This is unusual, but it has been known to happen.Some instructors are very "innovative", and I say that carefully because this isn't always a good thing.A few rare instructors have been known to run their classes more like a boot camp than a yoga class.They deviate from the true path of yoga in order to chase the almighty dollar by doing something "unique".But you can't get into the true spirit of yoga if you're being yelled at, degraded, and stressed out!

Yoga is about calmness, peace, and tranquility.It is also about discipline, yes, but not in a drill sergeant kind of way!The discipline comes from careful control of the mind and body by the individual, not by an outside source. If your yoga classes end up making you feel uncomfortable or upset, then you must question their value to you.When a class causes more stress than it eliminates, you should seriously rethink your choice to join it. Look for a class that looks fun and an instructor you like and feel comfortable with. The more at ease you are in the class, the more successful it will be for you.

Yoga Equipment

There are many items available for those who practice yoga. None of them are truly required, but there are many that would be especially helpful. You may have even seen a number of them in videos, on television, or in your local store. Perhaps you didn't even realize they were used for yoga. For many years yoga equipment was hard to find and somewhat expensive. Now it's very prevalent and the prices on most equipment are very affordable.

The problem is, the prevalence of equipment makes it hard to decide what you need and what you don't. You don't need everything, no matter what the salesperson may try to tell you. We're going to look at some of the most popular types of yoga equipment and accessories so you can decide what you need, what you might want, and what you can live without. If you're just getting started you really need very little, especially if you'll be taking a class.Your class may provide the items you need, but not all will.You'll probably need to bring your own mat at the very least. The equipment you buy will also largely be a personal choice.You may not need to buy something that someone else would consider essential.

For example, you'll find some people who prefer to sit on a hard floor or on the ground outdoors.Others find it very uncomfortable to sit on a hard surface and may feel pain in their back and tailbone.These people would really need a yoga mat.I'm going to simply describe each item and let you make your own judgments as to what is right for you.I won't try to tell you what you should and shouldn't buy, but I will tell you what I feel might be helpful.

Yoga Mats

For most people, a yoga mat will be essential.A lot of people won't be able to comfortably sit on the floor without a mat, and this can be very discouraging.You may be fine without one, but it's something you should consider.The first thing you should look for in a yoga mat is a good floor grip.You're not going to want a mat that will slip around a lot, especially while you're attempting difficult postures. You'll also want to choose a mat with enough padding to make it comfortable. You'll find yoga mats in different sizes, thicknesses, and colors, so you'll be able to find one to suit you.If you're going to buy one, you should be sure to find one that you're really happy with.

Yoga Towel

There are special towels that are made for yoga.You may find super-absorbent towels that will be quite helpful if you sweat a lot, and you may even find these in "chakra colors" which you can use in various situations. You may also buy a skidless towel that you can use on your mat to help absorb sweat. This may be especially important if you practice Bikram yoga.

Yoga Bags

If you buy a lot of yoga accessories you may want to buy a special bag to carry them. They look like duffel bags, and are often made of nylon. You can find these bags in many stores, and they range from around $10 up to $50 or $100.

Yoga Straps

If you have trouble holding your poses you might wish to buy yoga straps. They can help you hold those difficult poses longer.

Yoga Sandbags and Bolsters Sandbags and bolsters can help you keep your balance and support you through your poses. They come in many colors, and you may be able to match your outfit, mat, and other accessories.

Yoga Meditation Seating

Meditation seating comes in a variety of different types. You can buy special cushions, benches, and pillows for various poses, and they make it very comfortable for meditating for longer periods of time.

Yoga Balls

For around $25 you can buy a yoga ball.They help you learn balance, build your strength, tone your muscles, and make it comfortable for people with injuries to exercise. These balls provide extra support as you stretch, and are good for working out the back and hips, and can also be used during pregnancy. You'll need an air pump if you get one of these.The air will slowly come out of the ball as you use it, causing it to deflate after several uses, so you shouldn't forget to buy a pump to fill it back up.

Yoga Blocks

Yoga blocks are somewhat like mattresses.They have a number of uses, but they are most commonly used for body movement extensions.

Yoga Videos

Many people love to pick up videos they can use at home.They may not have the money for formal classes, or they may feel shy or awkward about attending classes with other people.Perhaps they just don't have a lot of extra time.Videos are a really good way to get into yoga if you can't take formal yoga classes.You'll be able to get in more practice and feel more comfortable doing some of the poses at home.If you decide later to take formal classes you'll already be a little ahead of some of the others in the class, especially if you start in beginners' classes.

Yoga Music

There are special CDs you can buy that are made to enhance the meditation experience.These can be used for enhancing the tranquility you experience. There are also CDs that help with your flow, including trance music.You may also find chants and mantras on CD that can help you get into the right frame of mind.

Yoga Clothing

You don't need any special clothing for practicing yoga unless you just want to buy some.Many people like to exercise in full leotards of different types, but a comfortable cotton t-shirt and stretchy leggings that breathe would be just fine.

CHAPTER 11: BASICS ON CHAKRAS AND HOW THEY RELATE TO YOGA

Our spiritual and physical bodies should be in balance in order to achieve an optimal experience while living on earth. This balance isn't realized by walking in a straight line or probably staying upright. It's facilitated by keeping the chakras open and balanced. You need to first understand the light that surrounds you in order to receive the energy balance in your entire body.

Though you might not know it, your body is surrounded by an energy that is constituted of various colors. This energy is sometimes visible in a clear and bright manner; in what is referred to as aura. The colors in your aura can change daily based on your feelings, mood or the mindset. In simpler terms, if you are holding pain or anger, your colors will be muddy or dark. The aura can remain dark until you fight or suppress the negative fear, pains or emotions. Then the energy is released into the universe.

Chakras are simple energy centers in our body. They are the openings for life energy to flow into and out of your aura. They serve to vitalize your body and to make you realize the self-consciousness. Chakras are connected to the mental being, physical body and emotional interactions. In case you block any chakra, you'll feel unwell and out of balance.

Let's briefly highlight the 7 common chakras, its color and its location.

The Root or Base Chakra

This chakra is red in color and is positioned at the base of your spine. The base chakra helps in tasks that relate to the physical and material world. In case the chakra is blocked, you might experience frequent colds, lower back pain, and fatigue. You can do the mountain and corpse poses to ground yourself and to open up the base chakra.

The Sacral Chakra

The chakra is orange in color and is located under the naval just in your lower abdomen. It helps connect you to the sensing issues that connect to your feelings. In case the spleen chakra is blocked, you can experience problems such as sensuality issues, urinary problems, allergies and asthma. Some yoga poses to open this chakra are child pose and twisted triangle.

The Solar Plexus Chakra

This chakra is yellow and is based above your navel in the stomach area. The solar plexus chakra helps balance the echo and intellect power. When the chakra is blocked, you can feel nervous; get diabetes, ulcers, and digestive problems. Do yoga poses like warrior pose I and II to open up this chakra.

The Heart Chakra

The chakra is green and is positioned at the center of your chest. The heart chakra helps monitor compassion, forgiveness, love or relationships. When the chakra is blocked, you can have problems like muscular tension, hypertension, breathing problems and heart disorders. Yoga pose like forward bend pose is effective at opening this chakra.

The Throat Chakra

It's a whirling blue-colored bright energy that is located in your throat area; and it helps to control your loyalty, trust, beliefs and to express yourself. You may have problems like infections, fevers, swollen glands and thyroid imbalance in case the throat chakra is blocked. Open this chakra by doing fish pose.

The Third Eye Chakra

It's indigo colored and is based in the middle of the forehead between your eyes. The third eye helps develop your psychic abilities and controls your insights and intuition. Blocking the chakra may lead to hormonal disorders, hyperactivity, shoulder, tongue, jaw, mouth and neck problems. Yoga pose like downward facing dog is effective at unblocking this chakra.

The Crown Chakra

The purple colored chakra is based at the top of the head and helps control your knowledge. The chakra also helps you trust the universe and control your dedication to divine consciousness. When the chakra is blocked, you'll face co-ordination problems, brain disorders, neuralgia, photosensitivity and headaches. You can practice corpse pose to unblock the crown chakra.

Here is an image showing how the 7 chakras are arranged in the body.

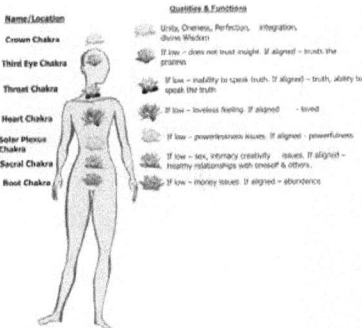

CHAPTER 12: DIFFERENT YOGA POSES FOR

WEIGHT LOSS

Yoga is a known stress buster, but it's also one of the most effective workouts for fighting stubborn fat stores, especially the ones that crop up after age 40. Yes, you can use yoga for weight loss. The reason: Studies show that yoga lowers levels of stress hormones and increases insulin sensitivity—a signal to your body to burn food as fuel rather than store it as fat. The following yoga poses for weight loss will do just that while firming up your arms, legs, butt, and abs.

Yoga has a number of incredible benefits, from decreasing stress and calming the mind to improving circulation and respiratory function. Many people think this ancient practice is all about meditation and flexibility, but it can actually be an extremely effective exercise for weight loss, and unlike a number of other fitness and slimming fads, it is extremely enjoyable and easy to stick to, which means you can keep the weight off!

Here are some different poses for weight loss

Crescent

Stand with feet together, toes forward, and arms at sides. Inhale and raise arms overhead, reaching fingertips toward ceiling. Exhale, and bend forward from hips, bringing hands to floor (it's OK to bend knees). Inhale, and as you exhale, step right leg back into a lunge (left knee bent about 90 degrees, knee over ankle; right leg extended and on ball of foot). Inhale and raise arms overhead; gaze forward. Hold, then return to standing and repeat, stepping left leg back.

Willow

Stand with feet together, arms at sides. Place sole of left foot on inside of right thigh, knee bent to side. Touch palms in front of chest for 2 breaths. On third inhale, extend arms up, fingertips toward ceiling. Exhale, and bend torso to left. Inhale and straighten. Repeat 3 to 5 times, pressing foot into thigh; switch sides.

Rocking Boat

Sit with knees bent, feet on floor, hands on thighs. With torso straight and head in line with body, lean back about 45 degrees, raising feet so calves are parallel to floor, toes pointed. On an inhale, extend arms and legs, keeping legs together. Exhale, and as you inhale, lower torso and legs 3 to 4 inches so body forms a wider V shape. Exhale and raise torso and legs. Repeat 3 to 5 times.

Hover

Begin in push-up position on toes with arms straight, hands below shoulders, and body in line from head to heels. On an exhale, lower chest toward floor, bending elbows back, arms close to body, abs tight. Hold a few inches above floor.

Chair

Stand with feet together, toes forward, arms at sides. Inhale and raise arms overhead, palms facing each other. Exhale and sit back about 45 degrees, keeping knees behind toes and abs tight to support your back; gaze forward.

Yoga For Stress Relief

Doing yoga for stress relief doesn't have to be an involved routine. If you don't have time to do a full yoga routine, use the separate parts of yoga to relax and rejuvenate.

Deep breathing, meditation and poses can go a long way toward conquering stress. Simple yoga techniques take minutes to do and can be incorporated into your exercise routine. You can also do them whenever stress takes its toll to regain your balance.

Try doing yoga for stress relief by doing parts of a full routine. If you are pressed for time, these techniques will fit into your life well.

Deep Breathing - If you want to instantly unwind and revive, do deep breathing. Most people breathe through the chest most of the time. This shallow breathing is caused by tension and stress. Breathing deeply through the belly oxygenates the muscles thereby relieving tension. Fill up your lower abdomen by breathing in. Contract the same area by breathing out. Do the breathing through your nose. This is the easiest part of doing yoga for stress relief.

Meditation - Spend a few minutes a day quieting your mind. It sounds difficult with a hectic schedule. Take a few minutes to sit in a quiet place. You can close your office door at work or go in your bathroom at home and lock the door. Sit comfortably and close your eyes. Breathe deeply and focus on the area between and just above the bridge of your nose. This is the third eye (eye of the soul). When a thought comes to your mind, envision it with wings and let it fly away. Do this until you are relaxed and centered.

Poses - Yoga poses are a sort of meditation since focus on the movements is key. Try these two simple poses to relax your body and mind.

1) Baby Pose - Sit on the floor with your knees bent. Make sure you are sitting on your heels. Hang your arms at your sides. Slowly lean forward at the waist until your forehead touches the floor. Rest your arms at your sides on the floor. Keep your neck relaxed and straight and breathe normally. Hold the pose for however long it feels comfortable - a few minutes, perhaps.

2) Butterfly Pose - Sit on the floor with your knees out and soles of the feet touching - like a butterfly. Keeping your back straight and holding your feet, slowly raise and lower your knees several times. Then, lean forward from your hips. Hold this pose for a few minutes while breathing normally.

If you don't have time for a full routine of yoga for stress relief, try deep breathing, meditation or poses instead. They are ideal for quick relaxation and regaining balance.

CHAPTER 13: YOGA WEIGHT LOSS POSES FOR THE ABSOLUTE BEGINNER

It should not come as a surprise to you that yoga is also a weight loss remedy. If you are wondering which poses to use when working towards gradual weight loss, I have you covered. In this chapter, we shall cover five of the most popular yoga poses guaranteed to help you burn fat and keep it at bay. Let us get right into it...

1-The Ardha Chandraasana pose

If you are afraid of strutting your body in a bikini because of buttocks, inner and upper thighs fat, this is the ideal pose for you. Additionally, the stretch also works on your tummy thus burning those extra love handles by strengthening you core.

How to:

To perform this pose, begin by standing with your feet together on your mat. Next, raise both your hands together over your head and hook the palms together. Extend out as if you are trying to reach for the ceiling, exhale, and from your hips, slowly bend sideways making sure that your hands do not unclasp. You should also keep in mind that you should not bend forward and your elbows should be straight. If you do it correctly, you should experience a stretch from your thighs to your fingertips, with the strongest stretch emanating along your back and the side of your stomach. The trick to this pose is to hold it for as long as you can and then inhaling as you move back to the standing position. Repeat the pose on both sides.

Expert tip: Do not perform this pose if you suffer from any digestive tract disorder, high blood pressure or a spine injury.

2-The Veerbhadrasana pose

The Veerbhadrasana literally translates into the warrior pose. It is ideal for stretching and burning the fat in your back, tummy, and buttocks as well as giving you killer thighs. The pose is also ideal for opening up your chest canals giving you better breathing. In addition, the pose is the absolute "mid-section fat burning Kung-Fu master."

How to:

To begin this pose, step onto your yoga mat. Place your feet together and place your hands by your sides. Next, extend the right leg forward with the left leg extended backwards. To get into the lunge position, bend the right knee gently. After this, twist your torso into the direction of your bent right leg. To get extra support so you do not fall, turn your left foot sideways around 40-60 degrees. Exhale and straighten your arms. Raise your body away from the bent knee. Next, stretch both the arms upwards and tilt your torso backwards (gently) to form an arch with your back. Hold the pose for as long as is possible. Remember to inhale and exhale normally. If you want to get out of the pose, exhale and push your right leg off to get back to the original position. You can also use your hands for support. Additionally, I would suggest that you take your time and be patient when performing this pose otherwise you may end up hurting your back, spine, or legs. Repeat the same for the other leg.

Expert tip: Do not perform this pose without the help of a qualified teacher especially if you suffer from joint problems or high blood pressure.

The Veerbhadrasana also has another variation; a continuation of the one above that is good for strengthening the muscles in your thighs, core, abdomen, and back. In this method, you begin in a similar pose as the one above but rather than raising your hands, you twist the torso to face sideways and then raise your hands to both sides in a manner that extends your fingers and makes them parallel to both your arms. Next, you turn your head until your eyes face the same direction as your hand (right hand) and then repeat this for

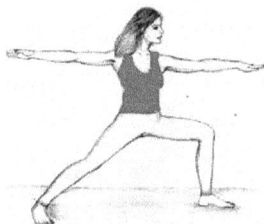

the other arm.

3-The Utkatasana pose

You may also call the Utkatasana pose the "chair pose". This highly concentrative and focused pose works on core strength, buttocks, and thighs.

How to:

Stand on your yoga mat, straight, with your hands stretched out before you. Raise the hands overhead and bend at the knee. You should make sure that the floor and your thighs are parallel. Then slightly bend your torso forward and breathe. Hold the position. When you feel tired and want to get out of the position, simply stand up.

Expert tip: This position is not ideal for anyone suffering from joint injury especially knee or back joint injury.

4-The Vrksasana pose

You may also refer to this pose as the tree pose. It is ideal for burning those love handles and giving you that flat tummy you have always wanted. It also tones your thighs, buttocks, and arms in additional to strengthening your core.

How to:

Get onto your yoga mat and stand with your legs together. Place your weight (most of it) on either on your legs and very little weight on the other leg. Lift the leg with less weight inwards towards your knee. You may use your hand to hold the ankle and pull the leg up into place. Place the heel of the foot you are holding on the inner thigh of the other leg making sure that it is as close to the pelvis as possible. When you get into this pose, you can let go of the hand and stretch your hands above your head and ensure that the fingers are pointing upwards towards the ceiling. In this pose, it is easy to lose your balance. Therefore, you should center your mind and concentrate on maintaining that pose. You can keep your concentration by focusing on one focal point and taking labored breaths. It is important to note that in most yoga poses, an unfocused mind will often times lead to failure and an unsteady body. Therefore, meditation is important so that you can have better control over your mind. While performing this pose, you should not hold onto a chair or wall for support, as this will reduce the intensity and effectiveness of the pose. You should simply try until the point where you can get it right each time.

Expert tip: If you are suffering from any back or knee injury, do not perform this pose without the help of a qualified teacher.

5-The Uttanasana pose

The Uttanasana is a forward bending pose that is ideal for stretching out the muscles in your abdomen and hamstrings. It is the ultimate relaxation technique because the blood rush to the head helps the body switch to the parasympathetic from the sympathetic nervous system.

How to:

Stand straight on your yoga mat. Move your arms in front of you and then proceed to raise them above your head while you take a slow breath. Bend forward as much as you can. This will force your buttocks to push back. You should make sure that your palms touch the floor and your forehead is touching your knee. You may find that you cannot do a complete stretch or the stretch feels uncomfortable on your hamstrings; in this instance, you may slightly bend your knees. Hold the pose for as long as you can and for as long as you are comfortable. To go back to the default position, take a slow labored breath as you raise your arms above your head while you raise your upper body. Exhale as you move your arms down from the level of your face. You should also remember to rise from the hips without putting any strain on the muscles.

Note: By practicing the above yoga poses, you not only burn fat, but you also tone your muscles.

Yoga Poses for Stress and Anxiety relief for the Beginner Yogi

We are all anxious and stressed at one point. Through years and years of practice, I have found that yoga works better than any power nap or cup of chamomile tea in reducing the stress. Let us look at some common poses you can try when you are dealing with stressful situations.

1-The Garudasana (Eagle pose)

The Garudasana is a balancing pose that helps the body move from the mind's distraction and towards healing and recalibration.

To perform the eagle pose, stand straight on your yoga mat. Next, entwine your hands together and place your palms against each other. Next, cross your right leg over your left leg and bend slightly. Hold this pose for 30-60 seconds and switch to the other leg. This pose is especially effective at quieting the mind and bringing the attention forth to the feelings of the body.

2-The Savasana pose (corpse pose)

This is the most logical position to get into after a long and tiresome day. It is ideal for relaxation and in essence, stress relief. To get into this position, lay flat on your back with both of your arms stretched at your sides. Now focus on your breathing for as long as you possibly can.

3-The Salamba Sirsasana (headstand pose)

This is the ultimate anxiety yoga pose. Why? Because by standing on your head, there is a reversal of blood flow. While the pose sounds and looks challenging, it is in fact not. To begin, you should perform the pose with the help of a yoga teacher or prop yourself against a wall.

4-The Viparita Karani (legs up the wall pose)

By using this yoga pose, anxiety becomes past tense. The pose does not demand that you be flexible, which makes it a style that even the beginner yogi can perform. To perform, simply lie on your back with your hands by your side and your feet propped straight up against the wall. You should make sure that your butt touches the wall. Now simply take slow in and out breaths and feel the nervous system begin to relax.

5-The Ardha Chandraasana (the half moon pose)

This is the go to pose when you want to cultivate a quiet mind and focus on what you are doing. This pose forces the mind to stop thinking of a million and one things and simply focus on the body, which makes it quite essential for stress and anxiety relief. To perform the half-moon pose, stand straight on your yoga mat. Bend to your left at the torso until your left palm touches the ground, then stretch your right hand upward towards the ceiling. After getting into this pose, stretch out your right hand behind you as high up as you can go making sure to keep it straight. Hold the pose for as long as you can and reverse it for the other side. You should also make sure that you inhale and exhale slowly.

6-The Salamba Sarvangasana (supported shoulder stand pose)

This is the ideal pose to be in when you are looking to experience something out of the ordinary. This inversion technique works best for stress and anxiety as it forces you to look at the world from a new perspective by yanking you out of your monkey mind. To perform this pose, begin by laying on your back on your yoga mat. Start by raising both your feet up above your body and continue by raising the rest of your body until only shoulders and head are resting on the mat. Place your hands on your upper shoulders for support and to prop the body, breathe slowly and concentrate on the breathing.

7-The Balasana (the child pose)

The child pose is the ultimate soothing yoga pose there is. It is ideal for an anxious yogi because it helps slow down the racing mind. To perform this pose, begin by kneeling on your yoga mat, and then proceed to sit down on your knees. Bend forward at the waist until your forehead touches the ground and move your hands backwards towards the soles of your feet. Hold the pose for as long as you can and breathe in and out laboriously.

CHAPTER 14: BODY AND BREATHING EXERCISES

Upon arising, don't jump out of bed rapidly. Take your time to stretch, bringing the body gradually to life again.

1. Stretching Exercise

Still in bed, flat on your back, do the complete stretching exercise. Start with one leg stretching slowly out, counting "one-two-three-four-five", up to ten, to begin with. Then bring the leg back and do the same with the other leg. Add one count every day until you count to 30. Stretching builds control of muscles.

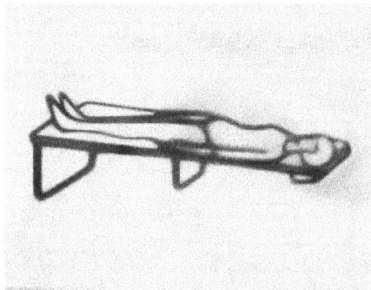

Figure 1- Stretching Exercise (lying on bed)

2. The Side Swing

a. Slowly get out of bed, first putting down one leg, then the other. Stand straight and continue to stretch the whole body (Figure 2 – A). Arms high above the head, swing to the left side and then to the right side (Figure 2 –B). Repeat ten times.

b. Stand with the feet apart, hands at sides, shoulder level. Start swinging the body from left to right, lifting the heel of the opposite foot, keeping the toe on the floor (Figure 2 – C). The head, eyes, and arms should follow the motion of the body with perfect ease and without any strain. The body and mind should relax with the rhythm of the swinging.

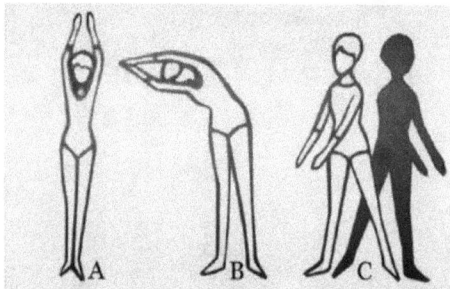

Figure 2 - Side Swing Exercise

3. The Side Swing to Floor

Stretch the arms over the head (Figure 3-A) and slowly begin to swing the arms from left to right, lowering them inch by inch, rhythmically and completely relaxed, until your fingers reach the floor (Figure 3 – B, 3- C, 3 –D). Start swinging back in the same manner with the same rhythm, bringing the arms to the original position above the head. Close the fists. Stiffen the arms, then let go, bringing the arms to your sides. Repeat twice.

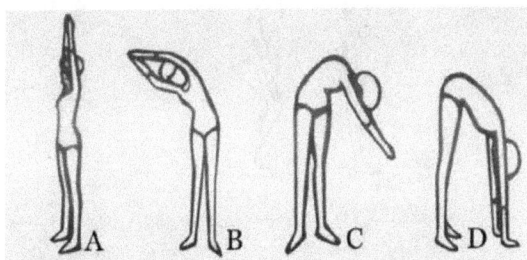

Figure 3 - Side Swing To The Floor

4. The Stomach Lift

Stand erect with the feet apart (Figure 4 - A). Inhale deeply, then exhale completely. Pull the abdomen in so that it becomes hollow. Bend the knees slightly and fall forward, hands on thighs (Figure 4 –B). Now pull the stomach in and out, doing it as long as you can while holding your breath without feeling a strain. This is one exercise. Repeat five times in the beginning and then increase to ten. This posture strengthens abdominal muscles and also helps to reduce constipation.

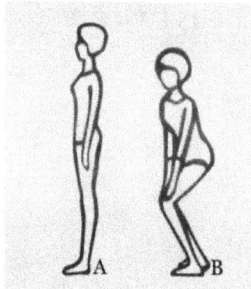

Figure 4 - The Stomach Lift

5. Exhaling Through Nose

The following rhythmic breathing exercises are done standing, feet slightly apart. Practice the complete yoga breathing, inhaling through the nose and exhaling through the nose, the mouth closed.

a. Inhale, rising up on the tips of your toes. Hold your breath while standing on your toes. Exhale while slowly lowering the heels to the floor.

b. Inhale, rising on the tips of your toes. Hold your breath while standing; exhale while lowering the body to a squatting position (Figure 5 – A). Stand up.

c. Inhale, raising both arms above the head, palms together (Figure 5 – B). Stretch. Hold your breath for a moment. While exhaling, drop your arms.

d. Inhale, bringing your palms together in front of your chest; hold your breath for a moment. Exhale, bringing your arms to your sides.

e. Inhale, hands on hips. Exhale slowly, bending forward (Figure 5 – C). Return to upright position. Repeat, bending backward and sideways (Figure 6 – A). Inhale and exhale each time.

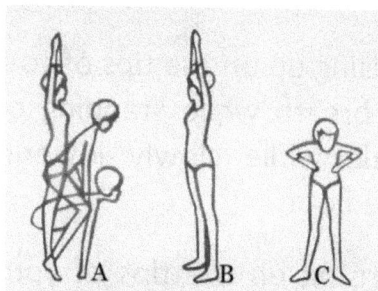

Figure 5 - Exhaling Through Nose exercise (A, B, C)

f. Inhaling, extend your arms sideways at shoulder level. Holding your breath, twist your body, arms sideways (Figure 6 – B). Exhaling, extend the right arm to the left foot, trying to reach the floor (Figure 6 – C). Return to upright position and repeat the same with the left arm.

g. Inhaling, slowly lift your arms above your head (Figure 6 – D). Holding your breath, stretch. Exhaling, bend forward until your fingertips reach the floor (Figure 6 – E). Repeat three times. Bending, your body should offer no resistance.

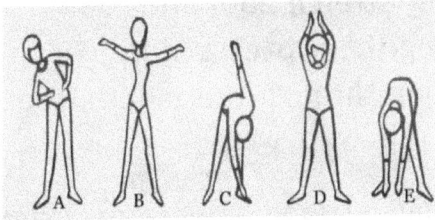

Figure 6 - Exhaling Through Nose Exercise (D, E, F, G)

Each of these breathing exercises should be done from three to five times. Each return to starting position counts as one. You can increase the number with experience, of course, but there are still other exercises to do.

6. Exhaling Through Mouth

The flowing breathing exercises are done standing, legs apart, inhaling rhythmically through the nose, but exhaling through the mouth in rhythmical staccato, forming forcefully a sound of "HA-HA-HA!" (This is known as a "cleansing breath" because it cleanses the respiratory organs.)

a. Inhaling, stretch both arms out in front, then swing them back and up (Figure 7 – A). Exhaling through the mouth, drop the arms.

b. Inhaling, stretch your arms forward, palms down. Holding your breath, move your arms sideways, lifting slightly in the shoulders, and forward again several times (Figure 7 –B). Drop the arms, exhaling with the mouth open. Exercises A and B are of great help in controlling nervous trembling of the hands or head.

c. Inhaling, place your fingertips on your shoulders and, while holding your breath, join your elbows on your chest, then move them wide apart several times (Figure 7 – C). Exhale through the mouth.

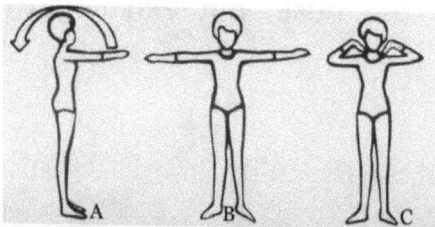

A   B   C

Figure 7 - Exhaling Through Mouth exercises (A, B, C)

d. Inhale through the nose in three vigorous sniffs. On the first sniff, stretch your arms forward; on the second, move them sideways; on the third, move them upward. Exhale through the mouth.

e. Inhaling, stretch your arms forward; hold your breath and begin to swing your arms like a windmill a few times in one direction (Figure 8 – A). Exhale through the open mouth. Repeat, swinging in the opposite direction.

f. Inhale, raising your arms forward, clenching your fists. Pull your arms back until your hands meet; hold your breath (Figure 8 –B). Drop your arms to your sides and exhale through the mouth.

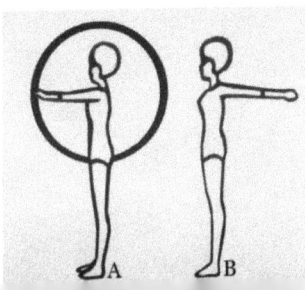

Figure 8 - Exhaling Through Mouth exercises (A, B)

Each of these exercises should be done from three to five times. Each return to starting position counts one. Again, you can increase the number with experience. The exercises described so far should take only about five minutes. If you have more time to spare in the morning, do a few of the vocal exercises and stop here. Other exercises can be done during the day. The relaxation exercises can be done at night before you go to sleep.

Chapter 15: Weight Loss And Yoga

You know yourself that healthy diet helps your body to keep in shape. You also know when you have over eaten or eaten food which isn't that healthy. As a beginner to yoga, you need to begin to take your diet seriously. That doesn't mean putting yourself on a limitation diet. It means respecting the needs of your body and eating the things that your body requires in order to be healthy.

Balancing your diet

Your body needs a varied diet which includes all of the vitamins and minerals that are needed to keep you in tip top shape. If you have decided that now is the time to commence yoga, you need to understand that weight loss can be achieved. This is achieved by understanding that your body is your temple and that what you feed it matters. It doesn't mean going on fancy diets but it does mean incorporating the foods which are in the food pyramid.

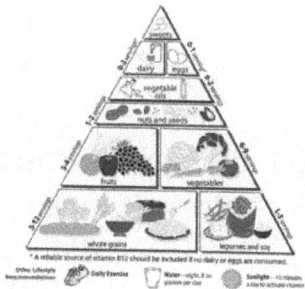

There is an extremely viable reason for the pyramid being the shape that it is. The lower portions of the food pyramid represent foods that you can eat in reasonable amounts, though don't overdo the bread! The upper area represents things that are not that good for you, such as sugars and candies. You already know this and the fact that you have chosen to take this journey into the world of yoga needs to be backed up with caring for your body.

The diet that you incorporate into your life should respect your body's needs. There are also food pyramids that cover all kinds of diets, so don't make the excuse that you are vegetarian or vegan as food pyramids also exist for most diets and show you the sensible quantities of foods that you should eat. If you do respect your body, of course you can lose weight and the exercise you get from your yoga will also help to address any imbalance that you might have which may be causing you to reach for comfort foods or eat the wrong things.

The importance of drinking water

The main complaint that people give for stopping a yoga regime is that they can't do the exercises. They may use the excuse of health reasons or of body cramps. What they may in effect be guilty of is not drinking sufficient water for their body's needs. Do respect that this doesn't include cups of coffee and tea. This should be fresh water and if you are not keen on water, add a wedge of lemon or a little flavoring to make the water more palatable.

Should I eat before doing yoga?

You should avoid eating for two to three hours before doing yoga. If your stomach is full then a sluggish digestion may be very uncomfortable. Eat light foods for the meal that you have prior to a yoga session, since the positions that you may use during yoga may upset digestion if your stomach is full. It's far better for you to change your routine, so that full meals are not eaten prior to your yoga class.

CHAPTER 16: THE YOGIC DIET

The practice of Yoga for weight loss is made all the more effective if you balance it with a yogic diet.This doesn't mean you have to give up any particular food group.It just means you will need to make healthier food choices.Cutting down on non-vegetarian food is recommended, though fish and other seafood can be eaten frequently.

Yoga encourages a largely vegetarian diet which is 'Satvik'.Food must be partaken of with care and regularity.Skipping meals is not healthy.Fresh, organically grown vegetables yield pure energy and provide you with all the nutrients you need.

Eat each meal at the same time every day.Avoid eating between meals.Try to cook your food yourself, using just enough oil, and never too much, and just enough seasoning to compliment the natural flavors of the vegetables or pulses that you are cooking.

Be aware of what you eat.Shop at organic stores or grow your own vegetables.Having a kitchen garden where you grow your own vegetables brings you into a closer relationship with nature and keeps you a happy, balanced person.Balanced mind= balanced weight.

Take a brisk walk in the morning to the local farmer's market and hand pick your vegetables.Choose vegetables that reflect nature's energy and vitality – bright shiny skins, plump flesh and crisp leaves indicate freshness and energy.

Use ghee (clarified butter) in your cooking, but never use too much.The Yogic way of life is one of balance, so include fats in your diet, but keep them in balance.Include dairy products in your meals, unless you are lactose intolerant.Even if you are lactose intolerant, the regular practice of Yoga will soon eliminate that particular health disorder, leaving you free to enjoy milk, butter, cheese, yoghurt and ghee.Eat as many vegetables as you can with the peel on, even potatoes, as this enhances their health value.

What to eat:

Fresh fruit

Fresh vegetables.You are advised to avoid garlic and onions, but this is not compulsory

Whole grains like rice, wheat and oats

All kinds of beans

Tofu

Nuts and seeds – preferably unsalted and in their natural form

Raw sugar

Plant based oils – sunflower oil, olive oil, sesame oil

Sweet spices rather than fiery, like cinnamon, cardamom, turmeric, ginger, cumin, fennel, etc.

Fragrant leaves like mint and basil

Foods that are not recommended

Meat of all kinds, particularly red meat

Junk food, foodstuffs containing artificial sweeteners, soft drinks...

Animal fats

Heavily fried or spiced foods

Food cooked in a microwave oven

Chapter 17: Mudras Therapy Hand Alignment For Holistic Health

The natural sciences of Mudra therapy believe that the five fingers correspond to the five basic elements viz. Ether, Air, Fire, Water and Earth.

Thumb – The fire (Agni)

Index finger – The air (Vayu)

Middle finger – The ether (Aakasha)

Ring finger – The earth (Prithvi)

Small finger – The water (Jala) So as to bring back the balance in the five elements, there are some specific methods of touching and aligning the fingers with each other.

These are referred to as 'Hast-Mudras' and this easy and doable therapy may be practiced anytime as an augmented relief from your malady as well as a handy tool for restoring your wellness.

149

Mudra Therapy: Hand Alignments for Holistic Health

Akash Mudra: For Ear problems

Dhyan Mudra: For Concentration power, Depression, and for all Mind related problems

Hridya Mudra: For Heart disease, Asthma, and Respiration related diseases

Jala Mudra: This is for blood purification and all skin diseases.

Prana Mudra: Eye problems, Nervous problems and charges all parts of the body.

Surya Mudra: Obesity, Cholesterol etc.

Vayu Mudra: For joint pains, stomach problems etc.

Prithvi Mudra: For peace of mind, Energy etc.

Various Types Of Mudras

Gyana Mudra

Joining tip of the thumb with that of the index finger forms this alignment. This is particularly beneficial for increasing the brainpowers of memory and concentration. Also recommended during meditation, this Mudra provides a soothing and calming effect to the mind. Those suffering from mental ailments like depression, anxiety, loss of sleep, stress etc may find relief on practicing the same. Not only this, in case you tend to remain angry and irritable in everyday circumstances and lose your cool easily, try this mudra and find the difference.

Dhyana Mudra

In this Mudra, you simply need to overlap your left hand with the right hand and keep steady in your lap. This alignment of the hands also tends to soothe your tensed up nerves. Practice this regularly to combat the everyday stress and strain and also for meditation. Varuna Mudra This Mudra is formed when you touch the tip of your little finger to that of your thumb. As specified earlier, the little finger represents the water element. Thus, the Varuna Mudra is particularly beneficial for dehydration. This may be also practiced for dry skin problems and it also works as natural blood purifier.

Surya Mudra

This mudra is news for all those who are evidently concerned about their expanding waistlines. This alignment has been particularly recommended for combating heaviness and obesity. For this particular alignment, you need to simply fix the ring finger in the root of the thumb and press the thumb over it.

Aayu Mudra

This may be rightly termed as 'Pain killer' alignment of the hand. The index finger is established in the root of the thumb and pressed with the thumb. Air or Vatta (being the root cause of pain in the body) is suppressed by the fire causing a reduction in the same. This is recommended for the patients of joint pains.

Prithvi Mudra

For those who feel the need to gain a few pounds and attain fullness in their body, this mudra needs to be practiced. For this, all you need to do is to touch the tip of ring finger with that of the thumb and keep the contact steady for some time everyday.

Prana Mudra

This mudra has been especially designed for attaining immune power so as to stay clear of body as well as mind disease. Also, it imparts a glowing complexion to the skin as it radiates blood-purifying properties. It is also beneficial for those suffering from eye ailments. For making this hand alignment, you need to join the tip of the thumb with tip of little and ring finger. Keeping other two fingers straight.

Apana Mudra

In this particular alignment, you need to touch the tip of your thumb to the tips each of middle finger and ring finger. The index finger and small finger should be held upright. Those suffering from frequent problem of abdominal wind may attain relief on practicing this mudra.

Linga Mudra

For respiratory maladies especially with increased phlegm and secretions, this mudra comes as help. It is particularly recommended for asthmatic patients and also for those who have increased 'Kapha' in their body system. All you need to do is to clasp the fingers of both hands together and keep one thumb upright.

Hridya Mudra

This mudra has been particularly designed for the heart patients. Patients of high blood pressure and palpitations may drive favourable results from practicing the same. The index finger is to be kept steady in the root of the thumb. Next touch the tip of the thumb to that of the middle finger and ring finger together. Keep the little finger straight up.

Shunaya Mudra

The middle finger is to be kept at the base of the thumb and the thumb exerts little pressure on it. This alignment may be tried at the time of pain in the ears. Those suffering from diseases of the gums may also benefit by the same.

CHAPTER 18: POWER YOGA

Moving to something with a lot more movement, power yoga is considered by many to be one of the best ways to lose weight naturally. Compared to Ashtanga yoga, it certainly is more vigorous and there are a lot more poses to keep up with. To help you get started, here are some of the most basic ones that you can easily practice at home.

☐Wind-releasing Pose: If you are looking to shed off some excess weight from your stomach or abdominal region, this is the pose for you. Simply lie down on the floor, your back flat against it. Slowly, lift your right leg upwards at an angle of 90 degrees. Fold it gently from the knee and rest it upon your stomach. Do the same thing with your left leg and hold both with your hands. Press firmly then release. Repeat the steps as you see fit.

☐Cobra Pose: This one is for working out the abs and the buttocks. Begin by lying down on the floor on your belly, resting both palms on either side of your chest. Slowly lift your upper body up, making sure your chest is off of the floor. Bend backwards as much as you can. Hold this pose for at least a minute before releasing.

Bow Pose: For toning your arms and legs, this pose is well suited for the job. However, beginners may find it a little tricky to do, so some practice is certainly needed. Start by lying down on the floor on your stomach. From this pose, slowly bend your legs upwards, from your knees. Arch your back as you do this and reach out behind you to try and take hold of your legs with both hands. Hold the pose for at least a minute before releasing. Do not fret if you can't do it the first time! Just keep practicing and you are sure to get the hang of it in no time.

Side Stretch Pose: This helps with increasing your heart rate so it's effective for burning calories. Since you are working on the sides of your body, it is also great for eliminating fat around that area. For this, you need to be standing straight with both hands on either side of your body, palms facing down. Slowly lift your hands upward, making sure to stretch them a bit as you do so. Once done, gently bend your body towards the right side. Stretch your right hand towards the right side of your head while you do this. Repeat on the left side as well.

☐Warrior Pose: One of the most popular poses when it comes to weight loss. It is great for developing and toning your thighs, arms and abs. It can also help in increasing your lung capacity. To begin, start on the floor and make sure your posture is straight. Slowly spread your legs far apart whilst turning your right leg in the right direction. Do the same with your left leg. This requires balance so don't rush. Next, raise your hands up and stretch them a bit. Join your palms together and turn your gaze upwards as well. Breathe in and out slowly to relax yourself.

☐Extended Side Angle Pose: Another pose that should help you get rid of excess fats from your sides. Begin in a standing pose and slowly turn your leg at an angle of 90 degrees. Keep your left leg straight. Now, slowly lower your body bit by bit. Rest your right hand over your right thigh, lift your left one up and stretch it over your head. Hold this pose for at least a minute before repeating it on the other side of your body. Do not forget to breathe in and out slowly as you do this.

Eagle Pose: Do you want thinner arms, legs and thighs? If your answer is yes, then you should be doing this pose. Begin in a standing position once more, keeping your hands on other side of your body. Slowly lift your left leg upward, folding it from the knee and gently wrapping it around your right leg. Again, balance is required so don't rush and don't fret if you don't get it the first time. Just try again. Once done, slowly lift your hands up, bringing them over your chest. Wrap your left hand around your right hand. Make sure your breathing is steady as you do this.

Pigeon Pose: The stomach has always been a problem area for many people and here is another pose to help you deal with flab in that region. First, kneel down on the floor and gently sit on your heels. Make sure to place both your hands firmly on the floor with your fingers pointed towards your body. Place your elbows in a way that presses them against your belly but make sure you do this gently. Next, straighten your legs from behind and slowly stretch. As you do this, lift your body up over your hands and legs. Your body and your legs should both be parallel to the floor. Hold the pose before relaxing.

Cow Face Pose: For this pose, sit on the floor and spread your legs out in front of you. Slowly bend them from the knees and place your feet flat against the floor. Gently slip your left foot underneath your right knee. This should place it right outside your right hip. Next, place your right leg on top of your left one. Don't rush as this requires quite a bit of flexibility and some stretching. After that, bend your hands backwards starting from your elbow. Stretch it gently in an upward direction. Your left hand's palm should be resting behind your back, right below the neck. Breathe slowly and hold your pose before relaxing.

Seated Forward Bend: For beginners, this is the easiest power yoga pose for weight loss. It is especially effective when it comes to getting rid of belly fat and helping you develop better abs. To get started, sit on the floor. Make sure your posture is straight. Next, spread your legs out in front of you. While doing this, exhale and bend your body forward from the waist and stretch until your hands reach the tips of your toes. Try to hold that position and stretch further. Remember, don't force it.

If you are unable to reach your toes the first time, you can gradually make your way to this with practice. Next, rest your forehead over the outer side of your knees or your calf muscles. Hold this pose for as long as you can, making sure that you breathe in and out slowly.

Benefits of Power Yoga:

☐ Known to flush out toxins from the body through sweating

☐ Can help heal problems such as acidity

☐ Burns more calories in comparison to other yoga practices

☐ Helps reduce the symptoms of hypertension as well as any issues when it comes to menstruation, including dealing with PMS

☐ Helps improve posture especially if you tend to slouch a lot. It can also improve your flexibility, stamina and strength

☐ Lacking concentration? Power yoga should help boost that.

Power Yoga Tips:

☐ If you're pregnant, do consult with your doctor before starting the practice. There are certain poses that might be difficult for you as well as dangerous so do take proper precautions.

☐ Practicing power yoga in the morning can benefit you throughout the whole day. It can boost your energy as well as your concentration, making sure that you are ready for the day's challenges. If you were nervous or anxious over something, it can also help you untangle those knotted nerves and take you to a calmer state of mind.

☐ Since you will be moving and sweating a lot, do make sure that you wear comfortable clothes for the practice. It should be something that will allow you to stretch comfortably and keep you feeling good about yourself even as you sweat.

☐ Don't rush! Understand that as a beginner, there are certain poses that you'll have trouble with. Maybe you are not flexible enough just yet or your balance is not quite on point. The key here is to practice regularly and make sure that you're following the instructions closely. Rushing might lead to injuries so do be careful!

☐Be aware of your breathing. There are instances when people don't realize that they've been holding their breath while doing certain poses. Breathing is important to yoga and helps your body relax even while you do strenuous exercises. Do make sure you keep your breathing steady and if you feel faint or out of breath, taking a break is an option too.

☐Lastly, do not overexert. Overexerting will not help you lose weight any quicker. In fact, you might find yourself injured if you push yourself too hard. Do everything in moderation and follow a slow and steady mantra for your practice. Take things day by day and you will soon see significant changes in your body and mind.

For people who want an exercise routine that would get their heart rate up but without requiring a visit to the gym, power yoga is one of the best options available. You can either enroll in a class or do it by yourself at home; what matters is that you practice it regularly in order to benefit from it.

CHAPTER 19: STRENGTHEN YOUR FEET

When you think of stretching a muscle, the opposite of that would be strengthening, right?Well, I have a few simple strengthening exercises that you can do with your feet as well.

My first suggestion is simple.Go barefoot Of course, one of the best things you can do for your feet is to simply go barefoot.When you are barefoot, all of your foot is being used.When you stand barefoot, your weight will be more evenly distributed.If it's not, then you will quickly notice if you are leaning to the side and placing more of your weight on one part of the foot.You will automatically shift to balance and have a more even distribution of your weight.When you have shoes on, it's not so obvious that you are placing more emphasis on the inner or outer part of your foot.A shoe will mask this because of the cushion that is built into the shoe.So, take off those shoes for a few minutes each day.

Many people have spent so much of their lives in shoes, that the thought of being barefoot is foreign to them.It might even be painful because your foot has gotten so weak.So, my suggestion is to just begin with small amounts of time.If you are someone who rarely goes barefoot, then start by just waiting 10 or 15 minutes after you shower to put shoes back on.Or maybe when you first come home, instead of changing into comfy slippers, walk around barefoot for a few minutes.

However, you fit this into your day, start small.Your foot will be weak and not used to the extra work that being barefoot will require of it.The good news is that even short amounts of time being barefoot will strengthen your feet.Over time, increase the amount of time that you are barefoot and start to notice how different your feet feel.

Feet really were designed to be barefoot.I like to think of them as masterpieces of design.You can move them in so many different ways, but over time with shoes on, we tend to lose some of that functionality.Going barefoot more often will begin to bring back some of the lost mobility into your feet.I know that most people don't have jobs where they can stand around barefoot.Being a yoga teacher does have its perks sometimes!I also realize that it's not practical to ask you to spend all day barefoot.What I am asking is that you kick off your shoes while you're at home a little more often.Give those feet a chance to breathe and move.Let those toes wiggle.Feel the freedom that goes with being barefoot.Try it and see how it feels!

Exercise:Take off your shoes and walk around for a few minutes.Notice your feet as you do so.How does it feel to have those feet come into direct contact with the ground?How do your feet feel with each step?Does it hurt to walk barefoot?Is one foot more flexible than the other?Do your toes flex as you walk or are they stiff?Try not to judge your feet or yourself for how those feet feel.Just be aware of how they are in this moment so that you know what you need/want to change about your feet.

Toe Lifts

Sometimes your feet are achy because they've spent so much time in shoes that they've actually become weaker.When your feet are being supported by shoes, they don't have to work as hard to adjust to the various surfaces that they would encounter if you were barefoot.Because of this, the muscles of the feet can weaken and get achy.

So, when I've had people asking how to make their feet healthier, I've often given them some foot exercises to do.Again, these same people come back and tell me how much better their feet feel.These toe exercises are fairly easy to do.They just take a little time out of your day and you can do them just about anywhere.You can also do them from a seated or standing position.

There are a couple of different versions that I'll introduce to you.Basically, these are exercises for your toes.Just like you can do exercises for your arms to make them stronger, you can also do exercises for your toes that will make your feet feel better.Here are the different variations for you to try.I suggest working with one foot at a time, but if you're feeling advanced today, you can do both of your feet at the same time.

Version 1

Let's start with the right foot.Stand or sit with your right foot flat on the floor.No shoes and no socks.Now lift just your big toe up off the floor. You want to keep the rest of the foot on the floor.I'm going to guess that you're not used to lifting just one toe at a time.Be patient.Let your foot figure out how to move in this manner.Repeat this toe lift for 10-20 times.You'll begin to feel it in the arch of your foot and maybe even further up your leg.That's okay.You're using your muscles a bit differently and they'll grow stronger as you practice this more often.

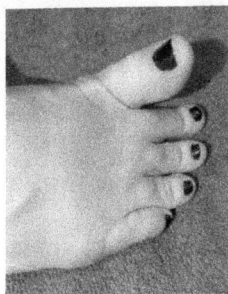

Version 2

Now for this second version, you're going to reverse the action.You'll keep the big toe down & lift the other 4 toes off of the floor.This might be even weirder for you to try.You might even need some help to do this movement.If you do need help, that's okay.You can use one of your hands to hold down the big toe while you lift the rest of the toes up.The rest of the foot stays on the floor.Again, do this 10-20 times for each foot.With time, it will get easier & you'll be able to do it without

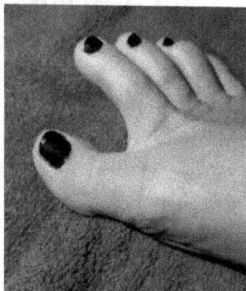

your hands holding the big toe down.

Version 3

I usually call this version the bonus round.You will keep your big toe down and your pinky toe down while you lift the 3 toes in the middle.Most people I show this to think that I'm a little bit crazy.You probably think that right now too and that's ok with me.I know that these toe lifts help your feet, and this bonus round version gives you the chance to improve your feet even more.Again, you can also use your hand to hold down the big toe and pinky toe when you first start to practice this.While you're lifting those middle toes, do what you need to do in order to keep the rest of the foot on the floor.It's ok to cheat a little bit.Your feet aren't used to this type of activity, but with just a little bit of time and practice, your feet can get used to this movement and get stronger at the same time.

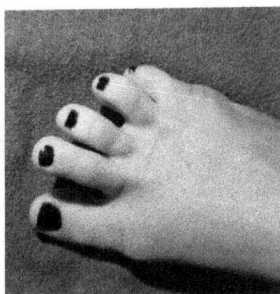

So how often do you need to practice these toe lifts?You can do them daily.It's a gentle exercise that will just make your feet feel better over time.Don't be surprised if your feet are a little tired after these exercises.They've worked more than normal!

Chapter 20: How To Master The Warrior Pose

"Virahabdrasana" or The Warrior Pose is an essential asana in any yoga practice. It targets the whole body with the legs, core and arms working together to create this beautiful, strong pose.

Begin at the top of your mat with your feet together and your arms by your side or in prayer position (palms together at the middle of your chest). Step one foot behind you, stretching your leg as far as is comfortable. You should be able to put your heel down on the mat with your foot at a 45-degree angle. Make sure that both your heels are aligned, keeping your front foot facing forward.

You are now doing the base of the Triangle Pose, but for the Warrior Pose, you will have to do a lunge. So, bend your front leg while keeping your torso upright. Try to get as low as you can, aiming for a 90-degree angle at your knee, although your knee should be found just above your ankle and not beyond it. Adjust your stance to be wider if this happens. Do not tilt your torso forward or backward; just allow it to remain in the same position as it would be in if you were standing up straight.

There are actually three different Warrior Poses differentiated by the numbers I, II and III.

In Warrior I, you extend your arms up over your head. You can put your palms together or just have them face each other. Your arms should be lined up with your ears while keeping your shoulders down. Do not shrug and aim to lengthen up towards the sky straight as an arrow while keeping yourself grounded on the floor. Hold this pose for ten to fifteen breaths. Afterwards, you can get out of the pose by lowering your arms, straightening your bended leg, and stepping the leg behind you back to your starting point. Do the same sequence with the other side to achieve balance.

Warrior II is similar to I, except for the position of the arms and torso. From the Warrior I position, you twist your torso toward the side that corresponds to the leg behind you. Simultaneously transition your arms from being overhead to being parallel to the floor. Just swing them down from their 12 o'clock positions to 3 o'clock and 9 o'clock respectively. Make sure that your arms form a straight horizontal line. Spread your fingers out and keep pulling yourself out to either side. Hold this pose for ten to fifteen breaths. You get out of this pose by transitioning back to Warrior I and following the steps outlined above. Repeat on your other side.

Warrior III is the most advanced Warrior Pose. From the Warrior I position, lift the leg extended behind you as you tilt your torso forward with your arms following. You are supposed to create a straight line from your back leg down your torso and your extended arms. When you are able to balance yourself, you may straighten your bended knee. You should be forming a T-shape with your body. Hold this pose for ten to fifteen breaths. You can get out of the pose by again reverting to Warrior I. Repeat the pose on your other side.

CHAPTER 21: KNEE PAIN

If you have arthritis in your knees, your knees are likely very fragile and prone to injury. When practicing yoga, this means you'll have to take extreme care to ensure you don't injure your knees further.

The postures in this chapter are meant to bring a gentle stretch, and sometimes even a challenge to your knees. Implement them into your routine with care. It might even be best to consult a yoga instructor and practice them under his or her supervision first.

When practicing these poses alone, have props like straps and blankets at hand. You should listen to your body and do not push yourself beyond your limits. A burning sensation in your muscles is normal, but any pain – especially a sharp pain – indicates that you should immediately and carefully exit the pose.

You may only be able to comfortably hold these poses for a few seconds and may not be able to enter the full expression of the pose. That's okay! Working your way up to these poses takes practice, but know that each time you mindfully practice one of these poses, you're doing your body a favor.

Wide Angle Seated Forward Bend

Sanskrit name: Upavistha Konasana

This pose provides a much needed stretch to your inner knees, thighs, hips, and ankles. In fact, it's considered one of the best poses for arthritis pain. It's also a deeply relaxing pose, so add this into your routine before bed or after a hard day.

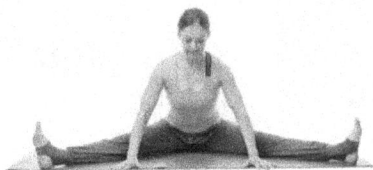

Instructions

Sit upright on your yoga mat with your legs straight in front of you.

Open up your legs as wide as feels comfortable. To give yourself more space, you may sit up on a folded blanket.

Press through the heels and activate your thighs.

Sit up straight, lengthening through the crown of your head, and then drape your upper body forward between your legs.

You may rest on your forearms or inch your arms forward as in Child's Pose.

Remain breathing in the pose for as long as is comfortable.

Props

If you cannot reach your torso to the floor, rest your upper body on a bolster, or support yourself with your palms on the floor.

Standing Figure Four

Sanskrit name: Ardha Utkatasana

Standing Figure Four Pose, also knowns as Half Chair Pose, brings a nice stretch to your outer legs, glutes, lower back, and of course, your knees. The standing version of this posture also builds muscles in the legs and challenges your core. Relieving arthritis pain isn't just about gaining flexibility; it's also about building muscular strength that helps to prevent injury further down the line.

If the standing version of this posture is too intense or challenging, see the instructions below for how to modify the pose to make it more friendly to your needs.

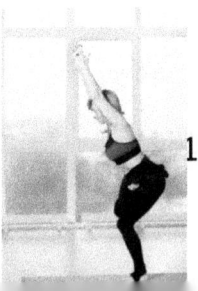

Instructions

Begin standing in Mountain Pose. Bend your right knee slightly.

Cross your left leg over your right, with your left ankle resting just above the right knee. Be careful not to cross directly on the knee, as this will put too much pressure on the joint.

Bend your right knee as much as is comfortable, until you feel a stretch.

Bring the arms upward with palms facing toward the body. You can also hold your hands against your chest in Prayer Hands.

Breathe in the pose as long as needed. Repeat on the other side.

Props

If you have trouble maintaining your balance, practice this pose behind a chair. Hold onto the chair for balance instead.

Modifications

If you are having trouble balancing, but would like to deepen the stretch, fold over your bent leg and place your hands on the ground, bending your right leg as much as needed to reach the ground. If reaching the ground is not possible, place your hands on a block.

For a milder version of this posture, try it reclining on the ground. Bend your knees so your feet are flat on the mat, then cross your left ankle over your right leg to create a figure four.

Warrior II Pose

Sanskrit name: Virabhadrasana II

Warrior II Pose is a foundation pose in the yoga canon. Most yoga classes will include this pose, so it's good to master it on your own. This pose delivers strength building to the legs and arms, while broadening across the chest, and bringing a gentle stretch to the knees and thighs. Because this is a more engaged pose, you must

exercise caution when practicing and be

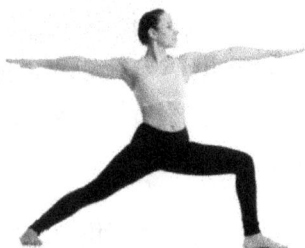

sure to not overwork your knees.

Instructions

Begin standing in Mountain Pose.

Step your right leg backwards on the mat about 3-–4 feet, depending on your flexibility.

Turn your right foot out at a 90-degree angle, but keep your left foot pointed straight ahead. Make sure your heels are in line with each other.

Begin to bend the left leg until it is bent at the knee at a 90 degree angle.

Stretch your arms out to your sides so they are parallel with the floor.

Inhale to broaden across the chest and open your shoulders. Check to make sure your shoulders are not tensing up and moving upwards towards your ears.

Activate your core and elongate your tailbone towards the earth.

Make sure your front leg is not collapsing inwards. If it is, this can cause pain or even injury in the knee. You should be able to see your big toe through the inside of your knee if you gaze downwards.

Turn your neck to the left to gaze over your fingertips.

Modifications

If you have a sore neck, look straight ahead. Do not turn your neck to look over your hand.

If you have sore shoulders, skip the arm posture. Instead place your hands on your hips or anywhere else that is comfortable for you.

Modified Bound Angle Pose

Sanskrit name: Baddha Konasana

Bound Angle Pose is a simple pose that brings a delicious stretch to the inner thighs, hips, and the knees. Unfortunately, the traditional version can be a little too much for some people's fragile knees. This modified version maintains the simplicity and stretching of the original while taking pressure off of the knees and hips.

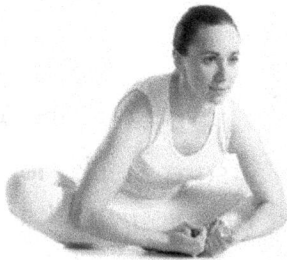

Instructions

Sit upright on your mat with your legs straight in front of you.

Bring your feet together so the soles touch and your ankles are resting on the ground. Then bring your feet as close to your pelvis as you can comfortably handle.

Place rolled blankets beneath the knees to bring some of the pressure off the joints. Lean forward from the hips if that feels good.

Breathe deeply to open the chest and remain in this pose as long as is comfortable.

Props

If resting on the ankles brings pain, place a towel or blanket beneath the ankles.

Modified Garland Pose

Sanskrit name: Malasana

Garland Pose brings a powerful stretch to your legs while opening up your hips. Not many exercises or poses target your ankles, which means our ankles can get pretty tight. Garland Pose is an exception, bringing a stretch to both ankles.

Garland Pose is also a relaxing pose that can help you to see big changes in your hips and lower body. However, it's not really ideal for those with knee pain. This modified version takes your knees into account, delivering a posture that can be done by those with sore and arthritic knees.

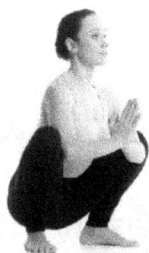

Instructions

Begin standing upright in Mountain Pose, then squat down. Your heels should touch the ground, but this isn't possible for everybody.

If your heels do not touch the ground, place a folded blanket beneath them.

To prevent knee pain, place a rolled-up blanket or a cushion behind your knees. Your bent legs will hold the blanket in place.

Bring your hands together in prayer pose with your elbows extended wide.

Use your elbows to spread your knees outwards and open your hips even more.

Breathe here for as long as it is comfortable.

Modifications

If the balancing aspect of this pose is too much, practice against the wall.

Extended Triangle Pose

Sanskrit name: Utthita Trikonasana

When it comes to poses that open up the entire body, Extended Triangle Pose might just take the cake. It's especially popular with pregnant women. This pose opens up your legs, hips, and lower back, while providing a gentle stretch to the knees and ankles, two areas that are so often neglected. It also opens up the chest and stretches the stomach, bringing relief for digestive discomfort.

Conclusion

Thank you again for downloading this book!

I hope this book was able to help you to understand what Yin Yoga is, and how to apply it to your life.

Body, mind, and soul share a very intricate and complicated relationship which make them inseparable. To experience the benefits of Yin Yoga emotionally and psychologically, you need to re-establish this connection.

This book gives you an opportunity to discover your life afresh and create an opportunity to lead a happier, more contented life. Through mindfulness, the core concept of a Yin practice, we can develop the potential to silence the non-stop chattering of our mind.

We come to an edge, surrender ourselves, and become still. We observe whatever is happening inside us, without adding any seasoning and condiments. We get the firsthand experience of what is happening in our life, right at that. With this new found clarity, we will be able to see the reality, beyond the false images that we have been seeing. We develop a sense of freedom that helps us to move forward by carving new paths.

The real benefits of a Yin Yoga practice goes beyond physical aspects. It helps us to create and establish certain good habits that we can carry with us till our last breath. When we learn to become aware of the present and enjoy this moment, we become free. And, when we experience this freedom, we become happier and independent.

There are so many wonderful ways regular Yin Yoga practice will enrich your life. You will realize that it is all about you. You now have to set yourself on this path to taste success.

Remember, reading alone will not do any good. Put whatever you have learned into practice. And, be consistent. Within a couple of weeks, you will notice and experience the wonderful difference!

Use the techniques and tips I have shared in this book and resolve to stay consistent with your daily practice. You will watch your life transform.

Best wishes!